POCKET BOOK

3

Endocrinology, Gastroenterology and Nephrology

Second Edition

D1392337

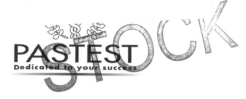

PASTEST
Dedicated to your success

MRCP 1
POCKET BOOK
3

Endocrinology, Gastroenterology and Nephrology
Second Edition

Colin M Dayan MA FRCP PhD
Christopher S J Probert MD FRCP ILTM
Timothy Heymann MA MBA FRCP
Helen Paynter MRCP
Julian R Wright MB BS BSc(Hons) MRCP

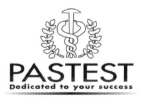

PASTEST
Dedicated to your success

© 2002 PASTEST LTD
Egerton Court, Parkgate Estate,
Knutsford, Cheshire, WA16 8DX

First edition 2002
Reprinted 2002, 2003
Second edition 2004

ISBN: 1 901198 94 4

A catalogue record for this book is available from the British Library.

The information contained within this book was obtained by the author from reliable sources. However, while every effort has been made to ensure its accuracy, no responsibilty for loss, damage or injury occasioned to any person acting or refraining from action as a result of information contained herein can be accepted by the publishers or author.

PasTest Revision Books and Intensive Courses

PasTest has been established in the field of postgraduate medical education since 1972, providing revision books and intensive study courses for doctors preparing for their professional examinations. Books and courses are available for the following specialties:

MRCP Part 1 and Part 2, MRCPCH Part 1 and Part 2, MRCS, MRCOG, MRCGP, DRCOG, MRCPsych, DCH, FRCA and PLAB.

For further details contact:

PasTest, Freepost, Knutsford, Cheshire WA16 7BR
Tel: 01565 752000   Fax: 01565 650264
E-mail: enquiries@pastest.co.uk
Web site: www.pastest.co.uk

Typeset by Breeze Limited, Manchester
Printed and bound by MPG Books Ltd, Bodmin, Cornwall

CONTENTS

INTRODUCTION

PasTest's MRCP Part 1 Pocket Books are designed to help the busy examination candidate to make the most of every opportunity to revise. With this little book in your pocket, it is the work of a moment to open it, choose a question, decide upon your answers and then check the answer. Revising 'on the run' in this manner is both reassuring (if your answer is correct) and stimulating (if you find any gaps in your knowledge).

The MRCP Part 1 examination consists of two papers, each lasting three hours. Both papers contain 100 'Best of Five' questions (one answer is chosen from five options). Questions in each specialty are randomised across both papers. *No marks are deducted for a wrong answer.*

One-best-answer/'Best of Five' MCQs
An important characteristic of one-best-answer MCQs is that they can be designed to test application of knowledge and clinical problem-solving rather than just the recall of facts. This should change (for the better) the ways in which candidates prepare for MRCP Part 1.

Each one-best MCQ has a question stem, which usually contains clinical information, followed by five branches. All five branches are typically homologous (eg all diagnoses, all laboratory investigations, all antibiotics etc) and should be set out in a logical order (eg alphabetical). Candidates are asked to select the ONE branch that is the best answer to the question. A response is not required to the other four branches. The answer sheet is, therefore, slightly different from that used for true/false MCQs.

A good strategy that can be used with many well-written one-best MCQs is to try to reach the correct answer without first scrutinising the five options. If you can then find the answer you have reached in the option list, then you are probably correct.

One-best-answer MCQs are quicker to answer than multiple true/false MCQs because only one response is needed for each question. Even though the question stem for one-best-answer MCQs is usually longer than for true/false questions, and therefore takes a little longer to read carefully, it is reasonable to set more one-best than true/false MCQs for the same exam duration – in this instance 60 true/false and 100 one-best are used in exams of 2 hours' duration.

Application of Knowledge and Clinical Problem-Solving
Unlike true/false MCQs, which test mainly the recall of knowledge, one-best-answer questions test application and problem-solving. This makes them more effective test items and is one of the reasons why testing time can be reduced. In order to answer

these questions correctly, it is necessary to apply basic knowledge – not just the ability to remember it. Furthermore, candidates who cannot reach the correct answer by applying their knowledge are much less likely to be able to choose the right answer by guessing than they were with true/false MCQs. This gives a big advantage to the best candidates, who have good knowledge and can apply it in clinical situations.

Books like the ones in this series, which consist of 'Best of Five' questions in subject categories, can help you to focus on specific topics and to isolate your weaknesses. You should plan a revision timetable to help you spread your time evenly over the range of subjects likely to appear in the examination. PasTest's *Essential Revision Notes for MRCP* by P Kalra will provide you with essential notes on all aspects of the syllabus.

CONTRIBUTORS

SECOND EDITION

Endocrinology
Colin M Dayan, MA FRCP PhD, Consultant Senior Lecturer in Medicine, Head of Clinical Research, URCN, Henry Wellcome Laboratories for Integrative Neuroscience and Endocrinology, University of Bristol, Bristol.

Gastroenterology
Timothy Heymann MA MBA FRCP, Consultant Physician and Gastroenterologist, Kingston Hospital, Surrey.
Christopher S J Probert MD FRCP ILTM, University of Medicine, Bristol Royal Infirmary, Bristol.

Nephrology
Julian R Wright MB BS Bsc (Hons) MRCP, Specialist Registrar, Department of Renal Medicine, Manchester Royal Infirmary, Manchester.
Helen Paynter MRCP, Staff Grade Renal & General Medicine, Gloucestershire Royal Hospital, Gloucester.

FIRST EDITION

Endocrinology
Colin M Dayan MA MRCP PhD, Consultant Senior Lecturer, University Division of Medicine, Bristol Royal Infirmary, Bristol.

Gastroenterology
Christopher S J Probert MD MRCP ILTM, University of Medicine, Bristol Royal Infirmary, Bristol.
Andrew D Higham MRCP, Training Fellow and Honorary Senior Registrar, Department of Gastroenterology, Hope Hospital, Salford.

Nephrology
Helen Paynter MRCP, Staff Grade Renal Medicine, Gloucestershire Royal Hospital, Gloucester.
Philip A Kalra MA MB Chir FRCP MD, Consultant Nephrologist and Honorary Lecturer, Hope Hospital, Salford Royal Hospitals Trust and University of Manchester.

ENDOCRINOLOGY

Best of Five

Questions

ENDOCRINOLOGY: 'BEST OF FIVE' QUESTIONS

For each of the questions select the ONE most appropriate answer from the options provided.

1.1 An 18-year-old boy presents to the Emergency Department for an unrelated condition and reports that he has a 'pituitary tumour'. Which one of the following most strongly suggests that this is likely to be a craniopharyngioma?

☐ A   He is being treated for diabetes insipidus

☐ B   He is being treated with bromocriptine

☐ C   He has been treated with radiotherapy

☐ D   He has received chemotherapy

☐ E   There is a family history of pituitary tumours

1.2 Which one of the following statements is most accurate regarding insulin-like growth factor?

☐ A   It circulates at levels ten-fold lower than insulin levels

☐ B   It is found at low levels in acromegaly

☐ C   It is found at low levels in starvation

☐ D   It is secreted predominantly from the neuroendocrine cells of the gut

☐ E   Like insulin it does not have a specific binding protein in the serum

1.3 An eight-year-old boy is suspected of having growth hormone (GH) deficiency. Which one of the following stimuli is the most appropriate to include in a provocative test for GH release?

☐ A   Arginine

☐ B   Glucose load

☐ C   Sleep

☐ D   Somatostatin

☐ E   Thyrotrophin releasing hormone (TRH)

1.4 **A 48-year-old man has hypopituitarism following pituitary surgery for a pituitary tumour. Which one of the following is most accurate regarding his hormone replacement regime?**

☐ A Adrenal replacement therapy be should started before thyroxine

☐ B GH replacement is rarely required

☐ C Mineralocorticoid replacement will be required

☐ D Testosterone replacement will restore libido and fertility

☐ E Weekly human chorionic gonadotrophin (HCG) injections should be used to replace luteinising hormone (LH)

1.5 **In a patient with suspected acromegaly, which one of the following is true?**

☐ A An increase in colonic polyps is an associated feature but these are not pre-malignant

☐ B A pituitary tumour can usually be seen on magnetic resonance imaging (MRI) scanning

☐ C A raised fasting GH level confirms the diagnosis

☐ D A raised prolactin level makes the diagnosis unlikely

☐ E Successful treatment results in resolution of the facial changes

1.6 **Which one of the following statements is most accurate concerning antidiuretic hormone (ADH)?**

☐ A It circulates in the bloodstream bound to neurophysin

☐ B It is a linear octapeptide

☐ C It is released by ethanol

☐ D It is synthesised in the hypothalamus

☐ E Its release is inhibited by carbamazepine

1.7 **Which one of the following is commonly associated with a diagnosis of diabetes insipidus (DI)?**

☐ A A requirement for urgent diagnosis and treatment with vasopressin in the central form (cranial diabetes insipidus) to avoid mortality

☐ B A serum sodium of less than 130 mmol/l

☐ C Autosomal dominant inheritance in the congenital nephrogenic form

☐ D Lithium therapy

☐ E Worsening with thiazide diuretics in the nephrogenic form

1.8 **A 23-year-old woman presents with galactorrhoea. Which one of the following is most important to consider in an investigation of this case?**

☐ A A careful search for an underlying malignancy

☐ B Exclusion of chronic liver disease

☐ C Exclusion of treatment with anti-emetic drugs

☐ D Exclusion of treatment with tricyclic antidepressant drugs

☐ E If associated with a prolactin level of < 5000 mU/l (normal range < 450 u/l) then an MRI scan of the pituitary is rarely necessary

1.9. **A 19-year-old woman with a body mass index (BMI) of 16.1 kg/m² is considered to have anorexia nervosa. Which one of the following is not consistent with this diagnosis alone?**

☐ A Elevated LH levels

☐ B Loss of axillary hair

☐ C Presentation with primary amenorrhoea

☐ D Raised cortisol levels

☐ E Raised growth hormone levels

1.10 **Hypogonadism in a 20-year-old phenotypic man may be associated with which one of the following?**

☐ A Anosmia

☐ B Complete androgen resistance (testicular feminisation)

☐ C Exposure to androgens in utero

☐ D Low levels of sex hormone binding globulin

☐ E Low levels of LH and follicle stimulating hormone (FSH) in association with the XXY karyotype

1.11 **A 33-year-old woman presents with hyperthyroidism and proptosis with diplopia and periorbital oedema. Which one of the following is most likely to be true?**

☐ A Antithyroid microsomal (antithyroid peroxidase) antibodies are likely to be present and responsible for stimulating the thyroid to overproduce thyroid hormone

☐ B If the woman becomes pregnant, transplacental passage of thyroxine may result in hyperthyroidism in the baby for several weeks (neonatal hyperthyroidism), even after the disease has been brought under control with antithyroid drugs

☐ C Levels of thyroid stimulating hormone (TSH) are likely to be in the normal range

☐ D Radioiodine may not be the ideal first-line treatment

☐ E The eye signs will improve with treatment of her hyperthyroidism

1.12 **In a 45-year-old woman presenting with profound primary hypothyroidism due to autoimmune thyroiditis, which one of the following is unlikely to be linked to the diagnosis?**

☐ A Addison's disease

☐ B Ataxia

☐ C Cardiomyopathy

☐ D Paranoia and delusions

☐ E Thyroid lymphoma

1.13 **Which one of the following suggests that thyrotoxicosis in a 28-year-old woman will resolve spontaneously and is best treated expectantly?**

☐ A Diarrhoea

☐ B Diffuse uptake on radioiodine scanning

☐ C Mild thyroid eye disease

☐ D Patchy uptake on radioiodine scanning

☐ E Tenderness over the thyroid gland

1.14   A 33-year-old woman presenting with palpitations is found to have a TSH of < 0.1 mU/l and a free T4 of 31 pmol/l (normal range 10–24). Which one of the following might best explain this pattern?

- ☐ A   Amiodarone therapy
- ☐ B   Normal pregnancy
- ☐ C   Occult abuse of T3
- ☐ D   Systemic illness such as pneumonia
- ☐ E   Treatment with interferon-α

1.15   A G-protein mutation may result in which one of the following?

- ☐ A   A non-functioning pituitary tumour
- ☐ B   Multiple endocrine neoplasia type 2 syndrome
- ☐ C   Persistent generation of cyclic adenosine monophosphate (AMP)
- ☐ D   Persistent hydrolysis of ATP
- ☐ E   Pseudopseudohypoparathyroidism

1.16   A 32-year-old woman presents with rapidly progressive hirsutism over the last four months, weight gain and muscle weakness. On examination she has clitoromegaly and a 'moon face'. Investigations reveal a raised 24-hour urinary free cortisol and an undetectable level of adrenocorticotrophic hormone (ACTH) on two occasions. Which one of the following is the most likely underlying diagnosis?

- ☐ A   An adrenal adenoma
- ☐ B   An adrenal carcinoma
- ☐ C   A bronchial carcinoid
- ☐ D   A bronchial carcinoma
- ☐ E   A pituitary tumour

1.17   Which one of the following is true of atrial natriuretic peptide?

- ☐ A   It causes increased thirst
- ☐ B   It causes salt craving
- ☐ C   It causes vasodilatation
- ☐ D   It is secreted by the juxtaglomerular apparatus
- ☐ E   It suppresses the release of aldosterone

1.18 **Which one of the following features is the best early indicator of inadequate glucocorticoid replacement in patients with adrenal failure?**

- ☐ A Fatigue
- ☐ B Hypoglycaemia
- ☐ C Hyperkalaemia
- ☐ D Hypokalaemia
- ☐ E Salt craving

1.19 **In an infant with homozygous congenital adrenal hyperplasia due to 21-hydroxylase deficiency, which one of the following is most likely?**

- ☐ A A female infant will present with intersex
- ☐ B A male infant will be feminised
- ☐ C Hypertension will develop in the first year
- ☐ D No effect will be apparent until puberty
- ☐ E 17-OH progesterone levels will be low

1.20 **Idiopathic hypoparathyroidism is most frequently associated with which one of the following?**

- ☐ A A good response in terms of calcium levels to treatment with calcium and vitamin D
- ☐ B Calcification of the tympanic membranes
- ☐ C Characteristic facies
- ☐ D Hyperthyroidism
- ☐ E Short fourth and fifth metacarpals

1.21 **With regard to Paget's disease, which one of the following statements is most true?**

- ☐ A Asymptomatic disease should treated be aggressively
- ☐ B Patients respond well to ergocalciferol
- ☐ C Serum alkaline phosphatase reflects disease activity
- ☐ D The disease is primarily a disorder of the bone mineralisation
- ☐ E The number of lesions normally increases over time

1.22 **Features of multiple endocrine neoplasia (MEN) type 1 include which one of the following?**

☐ A   Adrenal nodules

☐ B   Hyperparathyroidism

☐ C   Hyperthyroidism

☐ D   Hypothyroidism

☐ E   Phaeochromocytoma

1.23 **Which one of the following elements is most important in investigation of spontaneous fasting hypoglycaemia?**

☐ A   A sulphonylurea screen

☐ B   MRI of the adrenals

☐ C   MRI of the pituitary

☐ D   Thyroid function

☐ E   24-hour urinary free cortisol

1.24 **Which one of the following is of most value in the management of phaeochromocytoma?**

☐ A   Early treatment with β-blockade

☐ B   Exclusion of associated islet cell tumours

☐ C   Radiotherapy in the management of malignant disease

☐ D   Surgical histology as an indicator of malignancy

☐ E   Yearly screening with urinary catecholamines in familial disease

1.25 **Which one of the following statements is true?**

☐ A   Carbamazepine lowers vasopressin levels

☐ B   Desmopressin acetate has vasoconstrictive effects

☐ C   High gastrin levels are associated with pernicious anaemia

☐ D   In the absence of calcitonin, calcium levels rise

☐ E   The glucagon response to hypoglycaemia is exaggerated in long-standing type 1 diabetes

1.26 A 29-year-old primigravida woman with hyperemesis at 9 weeks of pregnancy has her thyroid function tests measured because of a resting tachycardia. These show TSH < 0.1 mU/l (normal range 0.4–4.5), free T3 6.8 pmol/l (normal range 2.5–5.2). There is no previous history of thyroid disease. On examination she has minimal non-tender thyroid enlargement. Ultrasound reveals a single live conceptus. Which one of the following is the most appropriate management strategy?

☐ A   Advise termination of pregnancy

☐ B   Commence treatment immediately with propylthiouracil with a view to dose adjustments through the remainder of pregnancy

☐ C   Commence treatment immediately with propylthiouracil with a view to performing subtotal thyroidectomy in the second trimester of pregnancy

☐ D   Withhold any antithyroid treatment and repeat thyroid function testing in three weeks

☐ E   Withhold any antithyroid treatment pending a radionucleotide thyroid scan to exclude transient thyroiditis

1.27 A 54-year-old man who has had trans-sphenoidal surgery and external beam radiotherapy for a non-functioning pituitary tumour six years previously has been seen by his GP recently, feeling increasingly tired with loss of libido. Tests done at that consultation showed testosterone < 0.1 nmol/l (normal range 10–30), TSH 2.3 mU/l. He now presents to the Emergency Department with vomiting. BP is 90/60 mmHg sodium 121 mmol/l, potassium 3.8 mmol/l. He is on no medication. Which one of the following is the most appropriate immediate course of action?

☐ A   Admit the patient for an insulin stress test to assess pituitary function

☐ B   Immediate treatment with intramuscular testosterone

☐ C   Immediate treatment with thyroxine

☐ D   Rehydrate with saline and then arrange a short Synacthen test

☐ E   Short Synacthen testing followed by immediate treatment with hydrocortisone

1.28   In the treatment of an acute asthmatic attack, β-agonists and corticosteroids are frequently used. Which one of the following is true of the molecular mechanism by which these agents act?

- [ ] A   β-agonists have a prolonged action because they act by both modulating gene transcription and an intracellular second messenger
- [ ] B   Both agents act quickly because they act via an intracellular second messenger
- [ ] C   Both agents act quickly because they have specific cellular receptors
- [ ] D   Corticosteroids act more slowly because they act by modulating gene transcription
- [ ] E   Corticosteroids have a prolonged action because they are lipid-soluble

1.29   In a hypertensive individual, which one of the following is the likely finding in a patient with renal artery stenosis and is helpful in distinguishing the condition from Conn's syndrome?

- [ ] A   A high aldosterone level
- [ ] B   A high renin and a high aldosterone level
- [ ] C   A high renin level
- [ ] D   A low aldosterone level
- [ ] E   A low renin and a high aldosterone level

1.30   An overweight 43-year-old woman is referred with the clinical appearance of Cushing's syndrome and a blood pressure of 170/90 mmHg. The best initial test to distinguish this diagnosis from simple obesity would be?

- [ ] A   An ACTH level
- [ ] B   An adrenal MRI scan
- [ ] C   A midnight salivary cortisol level
- [ ] D   Serum potassium and bicarbonate
- [ ] E   24-hour urinary free cortisol

1.31 A 60-year-old gentleman with type 2 diabetes has a myocardial infarction. He is treated initially with an intravenous infusion of insulin. He has an episode of left ventricular failure and is started on an ACE inhibitor. He has a degree of renal dysfunction with a creatinine of 147 μmol/l which is stable. He is usually on 80 mg bd of gliclazide. You notice that his Hb A$_{1c}$ is 11.2% and on dietician review there is not much that can be changed. Which one of the following is the most appropriate therapy for his diabetes?

☐ A Acarbose

☐ B Basal bolus insulin

☐ C Increase gliclazide to 160 mg bd

☐ D Metformin

☐ E Rosiglitazone

1.32 A 32-year-old man who has had type 1 diabetes for 12 years reports episodes of confusion occurring without warning. On one of these occasions, the blood sugar level on home testing was 2.5 mmol/l. The single best advice to help this patient for the future would be?

☐ A To eat every two hours

☐ B To eat less carbohydrate with each meal

☐ C To increase his insulin at night and reduce it during the day for three months

☐ D To reduce his insulin to maintain relatively high blood sugars (8–15 mmol/l) for at least three months

☐ E To test his blood sugar a minimum of four times daily every day

1.33 In a patient with diabetes and microalbuminuria, the most important element of management to preserve renal function is?

☐ A Aggressive management of hyperlipidaemia

☐ B Aggressive management of hypertension

☐ C A low protein diet

☐ D Avoidance of diuretic use

☐ E Improvement of glycaemic control

1.34 **In a 52-year-old man with acromegaly and a moderately sized (1.5 cm) pituitary tumour, the most appropriate first line of therapy would be?**

☐ A Bromocriptine therapy

☐ B External beam radiotherapy

☐ C Octreotide therapy

☐ D Trans-sphenoidal surgery

☐ E Yttrium implants into the pituitary

1.35 **Appropriate hormone replacement medication for a 28-year-old woman with primary adrenocortical failure (Addison's disease) would be?**

☐ A Dexamethasone 0.5 mg daily alone

☐ B Hydrocortisone 10 mg mane and fludrocortisone 100 µg mane

☐ C Hydrocortisone 10 mg mane and 5 mg pm, and fludrocortisone 100 µg mane

☐ D Hydrocortisone 50 mg bd and fludrocortisone 100 µg mane

☐ E Prednisolone 15 mg mane and fludrocortisone 100 µg mane

1.36 **In an individual known to have the genetic mutation responsible for multiple endocrine neoplasia type 2, which one of the following describes the two most important elements in management?**

☐ A Prophylactic thyroidectomy and bilateral adrenalectomy

☐ B Prophylactic thyroidectomy and regular pituitary imaging

☐ C Prophylactic thyroidectomy and regular screening for phaeochromocytoma

☐ D Regular thyroid imaging and regular screening for phaeochromocytoma

☐ E Regular thyroid and pituitary imaging

1.37   A 23-year-old woman presents concerned about increased hair growth. She is noted to have dark facial and lower abdominal hairs. She menstruates regularly but her cycle length varies from three to six weeks. Which one of the following is correct?

☐   A   A benign course is very likely in such cases

☐   B   Clitoromegaly is frequently observed in such cases

☐   C   If the diagnosis were polycystic ovarian syndrome, recent onset of hair growth would be expected

☐   D   Radiological imaging for a tumour of the ovary should routinely be performed in all such cases

☐   E   Testosterone levels would be expected in the low-normal male range in such cases

1.38   A 39-year-old man presents with a two-week history of polydipsia and polyuria. He is found to have a random glucose of 17.3 mmol/l. There are no ketones in the urine. He denies recent weight loss or vomiting. His BMI is 24.7 kg/m². Which one of the following is correct?

☐   A   He could be started on a sulphonylurea, taught to test his own capillary glucose levels and be reassessed in one month

☐   B   As in A but review in three months is more appropriate to assess progress

☐   C   He should be admitted to hospital urgently to commence insulin therapy

☐   D   He should be referred to a dietitian and reviewed after three months of diet and exercise therapy

☐   E   The optimal therapy is metformin

1.39   Which one of the following is true regarding carbohydrate metabolism after 48 hours of fasting?

☐   A   Amino acids are an increasingly important source of substrates for glucose synthesis

☐   B   Fatty acids provide 15–20% of the substrates for glucose synthesis

☐   C   Glucagon levels are rising

☐   D   Ketonuria is rare

☐   E   Liver glycogen is an important source of glucose

1.40 **A 23-year-old man is found on routine screening to have a cholesterol level of 11.3 mmol/l, a triglyceride level of 1.2 mmol/l and an HDL of 1.1 mmol/l. His mother died aged 45 of a heart attack. Which one of the following is most appropriate in this case?**

☐ A Excess alcohol is a possible cause

☐ B He should have a three-month trial of dietary advice before commencing lipid-lowering therapy

☐ C Treatment should commence with a fibrate

☐ D Treatment should commence with a statin

☐ E Undiagnosed diabetes mellitus is a likely cause

1.41 **A 64-year-old lady is noted to have a corrected calcium level of 2.85 mmol/l during blood testing for 'tiredness'. Which one of the following statements is most appropriate in this case?**

☐ A A parathyroid hormone level in the high-normal range makes hyperparathyroidism unlikely

☐ B A raised alkaline phosphatase level suggests bony metastases

☐ C Hyperparathyroidism and malignancy account for 90% of cases

☐ D If it is due to hyperparathyroidism, parathyroidectomy is invariably required

☐ E If the patient is asymptomatic, no further investigation is required

1.42 **Which one of the following statements about growth hormone (GH) therapy in adults is correct?**

☐ A It can improve patients' mood

☐ B It is currently associated with a small but appreciable risk of Creutzfeldt–Jacob disease

☐ C It is associated with weight loss

☐ D It is contraindicated in patients with pituitary tumours

☐ E It should be monitored with GH day curves

1.43 A 78-year-old lady is seen in the Emergency Department with right-sided loin pain radiating to her groin and the A&E staff report a capillary blood glucose of 9 mmol/l. On further questioning a history of polyuria and polydipsia is elicited, which one diagnosis below would unify these clinical and laboratory findings?

☐ A Autoimmune polyglandular syndrome type 2 (Schmidt's syndrome)

☐ B Primary hyperparathyroidism

☐ C Pyelonephritis

☐ D Somatostatinoma

☐ E Type 2 diabetes

1.44 In the diabetic clinic you see a 47-year-old woman of Caribbean extraction who has not been well for the last six months. She reports being extremely tired. She has lost 2 kg in weight. She has thrush and has suffered from recurrent urinary tract infections. Home monitoring tests (using a capillary blood glucose monitor) are mainly in double figures but the pre-clinic Hb A_{1c} is 7.3%. Which one of the following tests would best help clarify the inconsistency between the clinical picture and the Hb A_{1c} value?

☐ A Fasting blood glucose

☐ B HIV test

☐ C Renal ultrasound

☐ D Repeat Hb A_{1c} test

☐ E Sickle cell screen

1.45 You see a 42-year-old lady who has had type 1 diabetes since the age of 15. On her last visit to the diabetic clinic she was commenced on therapy for microalbuminuria but despite perseverance is plagued by a dry cough. Which one of the following is the likely culprit?

☐ A Atenolol

☐ B Captopril

☐ C Doxazosin

☐ D Losartan

☐ E Nifedipine

1.46 A 20-year-old lady is referred to the Endocrine Clinic with a six-month history of sweating and diarrhoea. She is otherwise well. Her father and grandmother died in middle age but she is unsure of the reason why. On examination, no abnormality could be found. Which one of the following diagnoses would it be important to exclude?

☐ A   Cushing's disease

☐ B   Graves' disease

☐ C   Growth hormone-secreting pituitary tumour

☐ D   Medullary thyroid carcinoma

☐ E   Premature menopause

1.47 A 24-year-old woman presents to her GP complaining of a sore throat, fevers, myalgia and a painful neck. She says she is very shaky and sweating more than usual. She has been having some palpitations. Thyroid function tests show TSH 0.1 mU/l, free T4 28 pmol/l, free T3 7.2 pmol/l. She is referred to the Endocrine Clinic. By the time she has her appointment she is much better. She has repeat blood tests which get lost but a TSH is done which is 9.6 mU/l. Which is the most likely diagnosis in the list below?

☐ A   Drug-induced hypothyroidism

☐ B   Graves' disease

☐ C   Post-partum thyroiditis

☐ D   Subacute thyroiditis

☐ E   Toxic multinodular goitre

1.48 An obese (BMI = 34 kg/m^2) 42-year-old man who works in a dress shop is referred to the diabetic clinic following failure to control his blood sugars on diet alone. He has been working hard at the lifestyle changes of diet and exercise. He has managed to lose 4 kg in weight over the last six months. The time has come when he needs further therapy to try to achieve good glycaemic control. Which one of these would be the most appropriate to start with?

☐ A   Acarbose

☐ B   Gliclazide

☐ C   Metformin

☐ D   Phenformin

☐ E   Rosiglitazone

1.49 **A 28-year-old woman presents with secondary amenorrhoea for 12 months. LH, FSH, testosterone and prolactin levels are measured and a Provera test is performed. Which one of the following combination of results would be most consistent with a diagnosis of polycystic ovarian syndrome?**

☐ A   A high FSH (> 20 U/l) and a mildly raised prolactin

☐ B   A high FSH (> 20 U/l) and an undetectable testosterone level

☐ C   A moderately raised LH and no withdrawal bleed following Provera challenge

☐ D   A moderately raised LH level and a positive withdrawal bleed following Provera challenge

☐ E   Undetectable LH and FSH levels and a raised prolactin

1.50 **A 30-year-old woman with maturity-onset diabetes of the young presents to the diabetic clinic because she is 12 weeks pregnant. Her glycaemic control is excellent with an Hb A_{1c} of 5.7% on gliclazide 80 mg bd. How would you manage her?**

☐ A   Change gliclazide to glibenclamide

☐ B   Continue present management

☐ C   Increase gliclazide to 160 mg bd

☐ D   Replace gliclazide with basal bolus insulin

☐ E   Replace gliclazide with Mixtard insulin bd

GASTROENTEROLOGY

Best of Five

Questions

GASTROENTEROLOGY: 'BEST OF FIVE' QUESTIONS

For each of the questions select the ONE most appropriate answer from the options provided.

2.1 **Which one of the following methods is the single most effective way to induce and maintain gastric achlorhydria?**

☐ A Administer a continuous nasogastric infusion of an antacid such as magnesium trisilicate mixture

☐ B Administer high-dose intravenous proton pump inhibitors (PPIs)

☐ C Cut the vagus nerve

☐ D Introduce *Helicobacter pylori* infection

☐ E Perform a partial gastrectomy

2.2 **A 74-year-old woman is referred with a history of pruritis and lethargy that dates back many months. She has abnormal liver function tests, total bilirubin 43 mmol/l, alanine aminotransferase 58 U/l, alkaline phosphatase 412 U/l, albumin 34 g/l. An abdominal ultrasound scan shows no evidence of bile duct obstruction or obvious liver disease. Subsequently, you find she has a positive antimitochondrial antibody result. Her liver biopsy histology shows periportal fibrosis and inflammation. You tell her that she has primary biliary cirrhosis. Which one of the following is most accurate?**

☐ A As the pruritis is due to raised circulating bilirubin levels, bile salt-binding agents such as cholestyramine are likely to give symptom relief

☐ B Because primary biliary cirrhosis is an autoimmune disease, oral steroids are likely to be helpful

☐ C Given her age, the disease is unlikely to affect her life expectancy

☐ D Serum bilirubin levels can be used to determine the optimum timing for possible orthotopic liver transplantation but are unhelpful if the patient has been taking ursodeoxycholic acid

☐ E Ursodeoxycholic acid will help her symptoms and may delay disease progression

2.3 A young woman is brought into hospital as an emergency by ambulance. She had been found, drowsy, by her boyfriend on his return home from work that evening. He tells you that they had had a row that morning. He had found an empty packet of paracetamol tablets in the kitchen. You make a rapid clinical assessment of the patient and note her stable observations but depressed Glasgow Coma Scale score of 13/15. You obtain a venous blood sample to send to the laboratory for tests. Which one of the following would be your next priority?

- ☐ A Arrange urgent gastric lavage
- ☐ B Ask the nursing staff to monitor her blood glucose levels
- ☐ C Contact your regional liver unit as the patient has clearly taken a significant overdose and may need transfer
- ☐ D Seek psychiatric input
- ☐ E Start an *N*-acetylcysteine infusion

2.4 A retired man presents with tingling in his hands and feet. He admits to having a poor appetite and modest weight loss over the past year though you find it difficult to keep him focused on the consultation. On clinical examination you are struck by his pallor and the beefy appearance of his tongue. He also appears to have paraesthesiae in a 'glove and stocking' distribution and muscle wasting. You are not surprised to find a macrocytosis on his blood film. Which is the most likely explanation for his presentation?

- ☐ A Chronic pancreatitis
- ☐ B Coeliac disease
- ☐ C His use of over-the-counter vitamin C preparations
- ☐ D Inadequate diet
- ☐ E Pernicious anaemia

2.5 **The report from your patient's recent elective oesophagogastro-duodenoscopy comments on an incidental finding of prominent oesophageal varices. In addition to the need to determine the cause for the varices, further management should include which one of the following?**

- ☐ A   Serial endoscopy and banding of varices until the varices have been eradicated
- ☐ B   Serial endoscopy and variceal sclerotherapy until the varices have been eradicated
- ☐ C   The regular use of a vasopressin analogue such as terlipressin to maintain portal pressure below 12 mmHg
- ☐ D   The use of a non-selective β-blocker such as propanolol to maintain portal pressure below 12 mmHg
- ☐ E   The use of a selective β-blocker such as atenolol to maintain portal pressure below 15 mmHg

2.6 **Which one of the following reasons best explains why population screening for colorectal cancer may be introduced in the United Kingdom?**

- ☐ A   Beer drinking is very popular
- ☐ B   Colorectal cancer is a more common cause of cancer death than cervical cancer
- ☐ C   Consumption of red meat and animal fat has been rising steadily with increasing prosperity
- ☐ D   It is likely to be at least as cost-effective as screening for cervical cancer
- ☐ E   Newer faecal occult blood testing methods are increasingly sensitive and specific

2.7 **Acquired immunodeficiency may be associated with several gastrointestinal and liver disorders. Which one of the following would be least likely to be associated with advanced HIV infection?**

- ☐ A   Anal tumours
- ☐ B   Chronic hepatitis C infection
- ☐ C   *Cryptosporidium*-associated diarrhoea
- ☐ D   Hepatitis B surface antigen-positive status
- ☐ E   Troublesome perianal Crohn's disease

2.8   A 76-year-old man presents with chronic central abdominal pain. He
       reports that his stool has become looser in the last few days. He drinks
       little alcohol and although he has felt somewhat nauseated with the pain he
       denies any weight loss. He has been taking the non-steroidal anti-
       inflammatory drug (NSAID) diclofenac for back pain. More recently his GP
       has given him a PPI (lansoprazole) which has helped somewhat.
       Nevertheless, he remains aware of discomfort in the abdomen. Clinical
       examination adds little. Investigations for which his GP had sent him have
       shown a normal full blood count, urea and electrolytes, liver function tests,
       serum amylase and serum calcium. He is positive for *Helicobacter pylori*
       IgG (immunoglobulin G). Which of the following statements is accurate?

☐ A   Colonoscopy would be a more useful next investigation than
       oesophagogastroduodenoscopy given the change of bowel habit

☐ B   His GP may have been better advised to refer the patient for
       oesophagogastroduodenoscopy rather than test for *H. pylori* serology

☐ C   *H. pylori* eradication therapy should have been tried before referral to
       hospital

☐ D   The *H. pylori* result is likely to reflect past infection only

☐ E   The patient's *H. pylori* status should have been checked before starting
       him on NSAIDs

2.9   You have invited a friend with coeliac disease round for dinner. You have
       decided what you are going to eat and drink. You have taken care to
       remove pasta and cakes from the menu but then realise that you may be
       drinking alone. Which one of the following had you planned to serve?

☐ A   A low-alcohol lager

☐ B   Cranberry juice

☐ C   Gin and tonic

☐ D   Green tea

☐ E   White wine

2.10 Every week a district nurse has been visiting an 80-year-old woman at home to dress chronic leg ulcers. Two weeks ago he had felt that the ulcers had become infected. In consultation with the patient's GP he has decided to start treatment with the antibiotic metronidazole. He was unable to visit last week but on his return earlier today he discovered that the woman had developed the most appalling diarrhoea. The patient had also become somewhat confused. She appeared dehydrated, pulse 86 bpm and temperature 37.6 °C. The nurse observed traces of bright blood in the toilet. What advice would you give to him?

☐ A It would be reasonable to stop the antibiotic, give Dioralyte (an oral rehydration salt) and review the patient in 72 hours

☐ B She must be sent to hospital as she is confused

☐ C She must be sent to hospital as she is dehydrated and pyrexial: given the history you are concerned to diagnose and treat any antibiotic-associated complications as soon as possible

☐ D She must be sent to hospital for further assessment as she is dehydrated and pyrexial, although pseudomembranous colitis can be discounted as the cause as metronidazole is used as treatment for this condition – it does not cause it

☐ E You feel that ischaemic colitis seems most likely given her chronic leg ulceration. In additon, your records show that she has been an inpatient recently and was successfully treated for *Clostridium difficile*-associated colitis. Relapse is very uncommon after treatment

2.11 A 40-year-old lawyer in whom you have recently diagnosed alcohol-induced chronic pancreatitis returns to see you to review treatment options. Which one of the following are you able to tell her?

☐ A Her prognosis is better if she abstains from alcohol permanently

☐ B Her prognosis is good provided that she does not smoke

☐ C Pancreatectomy should be performed early in the course of the disease

☐ D The duration of any relapse will become shorter as the pancreas burns itself out over time

☐ E The use of pancreatic enzyme supplements will improve both her symptoms and her prognosis

2.12   A 32-year-old woman attends your surgery to discuss her dietary needs ahead of a planned pregnancy. She is concerned that, as she has had surgery for small bowel Crohn's disease some years ago, the general advice offered about folic acid supplementation may not be appropriate for her. Unfortunately, your records do not confirm what operation was performed. Which of the following is most accurate?

☐ A   As signs and symptoms of folate deficiency typically take four months to manifest themselves, and if her serum and red cell folate levels are satisfactory ahead of conception, she need not worry about taking folate supplements. The risk to the fetus of developing neural tube problems arises only in the first trimester of pregnancy

☐ B   If her operation for Crohn's disease has left her with a blind loop, bacteria may be competing for her dietary folate so supplementation at a higher than normal dose may be sensible

☐ C   If she has had her small bowel resected she may be malabsorbing folic acid and so supplementation at a higher than normal dose would be advised

☐ D   She may follow normal advice on supplementation (folic acid 400 mg daily) but should also cook her food thoroughly to improve the bioavailability of dietary folate

☐ E   She should ensure that her diet is rich in foods that contain folate, such as nuts, liver and green vegetables

2.13   A 60-year-old executive presents with confusion. You had met him some months previously when he had ascites. A diagnosis of alcohol-induced cirrhotic liver disease was made. On this occasion you note stigmata of chronic liver disease, including spider naevi and mild gynaecomastia. You find no ascites but mild peripheral oedema. His blood profile shows a mild hyponatraemia (perhaps a consequence of the diuretics which you had started him on), a serum albumin of 22 g/l and liver function tests show an international normalised ratio (INR) of 2.1. Your view that his confusion reflects a hepatic encephalopathy is supported by which one of the following?

☐ A   An absent pupillary response

☐ B   An associated headache

☐ C   His family's description of an inversion of his normal sleep pattern

☐ D   His inability to recall either the name of the Queen or the Prime Minister

☐ E   Your clinical finding of hyporeflexia

2.14 **A 29-year-old woman presents with an incidental finding of a mild iron deficiency anaemia. Menstruation-associated blood loss, dietary insufficiency and malabsorption have been excluded by others. Indeed, the latter would have been very surprising as you understand that she suffers from constipation rather than diarrhoea. She also admits to bright-red rectal bleeding and has been putting on weight. At flexible sigmoidoscopy you only find a discrete area of ulcerated anterior rectal mucosa. You take biopsies from the area but meanwhile you should do which one of the following?**

  □ A Consider that your findings are not adequate to explain her anaemia

  □ B Express surprise at finding what appears to be a solitary rectal ulcer in a young woman

  □ C Express surprise that the ulcer is sited anteriorly

  □ D Offer advice on laxatives

  □ E Offer to start the patient on mesalazine suppositories

2.15 **Which of the following is true regarding cholecystokinin?**

  □ A In excess, it precipitates gallstones

  □ B It causes delayed gastric emptying through its action as a smooth muscle relaxant

  □ C It is found in higher concentrations following cholecystectomy

  □ D It releases the 'ileal brake'

  □ E It stimulates pancreatic exocrine secretion

2.16   A 34-year-old Foreign Office employee has spent much of his early career in South America. He is used to stomach upsets but following his return from a posting in Brazil about 15 months ago he reports that his bowel habit has been very erratic although it does not disturb him at night. His stools may be mushy or look like 'runner beans'. He reports no weight loss nor has he observed any rectal bleeding. His stools flush away. He has an associated vague abdominal pain that improves once he has opened his bowels but he never feels that his bowel is 'empty'. Clinical examination, including rigid sigmoidoscopy, baseline blood tests and laboratory investigation of his stools all fail to identify any abnormality. Which one of the following is the most appropriate statement?

☐ A   As he has been working in South America, investigation for tropical disease is necessary

☐ B   As he is colour blind it would be unsafe to make a diagnosis of irritable bowel syndrome until faecal occult blood tests are confirmed as negative

☐ C   'Runner bean' stools are characteristic of conditions causing colonic stricture

☐ D   The patient has Chagas' disease

☐ E   The patient has irritable bowel syndrome

2.17   A 19-year-old man of Japanese extraction presents with haematemesis. Despite the language barrier you ascertain that he drinks little alcohol but has recently started to take drugs for a psychiatric illness. On clinical examination you find stigmata of chronic liver disease. You go on to perform upper GI endoscopy and find bleeding oesophageal varices that you treat successfully with banding. Further imaging is in keeping with cirrhosis with portal hypertension and extensive collaterals. His liver function tests are only mildly deranged (INR = 1.4). You send off a liver screen to determine the cause. The laboratory reports only a low serum caeruloplasmin level, suggesting that he has Wilson's disease. Which one of the following is the most appropriate statement in this case?

☐ A   He should be listed for liver transplantation

☐ B   Kayser–Fleischer rings are likely to be absent given that he has psychiatric manifestations of the disease

☐ C   Liver biopsy must be done as the next step

☐ D   The diagnosis is especially surprising given the patient's ethnicity

☐ E   Treatment with penicillamine and zinc should be started

2.18 You receive the following blood test results from a 58-year-old Cypriot woman: serum bilirubin 40 mmol/l, alanine aminotransferase 23 U/l, alkaline phosphatase 80 U/l, serum albumin 36 g/l, haemoglobin 127 g/l, mean corpuscular volume (MCV) 80 fl, platelet count 360×10^9/l. Her family comments that she often looks a little yellow. In herself she feels well. Which one of the following statements is correct?

- [ ] A   Her liver function tests need to be carefully monitored
- [ ] B   Most of the bilirubin is likely to be bound to albumin
- [ ] C   Most of the bilirubin is likely to be conjugated
- [ ] D   One in four of her siblings is likely to have a similar problem
- [ ] E   The findings are compatible with primary biliary cirrhosis

2.19 A 65-year-old man is referred to you with abnormal liver function tests: alanine aminotransferase 85 U/l, alkaline phosphatase150 U/l, albumin 36 g/l, bilirubin 14 mmol/l. They had been noticed as part of a well-man screen. In himself he is well. On taking a detailed medical history you can identify no potential cause for liver disease. Indeed, the patient had been so fit and well that he was a regular blood donor up to the age of 60. Clinical examination identifies no abnormality. You send off a screen for the normal causes of liver disease, including viral serology, an autoimmune profile and a serum ferritin level. Only the latter is raised sixfold. Which one of the following should be your next priority?

- [ ] A   Alert the blood transfusion service
- [ ] B   Organise a liver biopsy
- [ ] C   Recommend venesection pending other investigations, all of which will take time to arrange
- [ ] D   Send blood for genetic studies looking for mutations of the haemochromatosis gene (*HFE*)
- [ ] E   Suggest members of his family are screened

2.20   **A member of the national rugby team comes to consult you. He has become increasingly concerned by symptoms of heartburn and waterbrash, especially after training sessions in the gym. While his symptoms respond promptly to the antacids that he has taken almost daily for several years, he wonders whether any investigations should be done and whether more effective treatments exist. Which one of the following statements is true?**

   ☐ A   Endoscopy is needed to confirm the diagnosis of gastro oesophageal reflux disease

   ☐ B   Endoscopy is needed to rule out other disease

   ☐ C   Oesophageal pH and manometry studies are required

   ☐ D   Reflux following physical activity is a common problem and as long as the antacids work nothing more needs to be done

   ☐ E   You should prescribe an H_2-receptor antagonist such as ranitidine for him

2.21   **A 32-year-old pilot presents with pain and difficulty on swallowing. Her GP, who had recently diagnosed Raynaud's phenomenon and started her on the calcium channel blocker nifedipine, postulates that the dysphagia may be stress-related as her fitness to fly was due for review. A trial of PPIs has not really helped. Which one of the following statements offers the most appropriate action?**

   ☐ A   You agree with the GP and reassure the patient accordingly

   ☐ B   You arrange upper GI tract endoscopy

   ☐ C   You consider that a trial period off nifedipine would help as that drug relaxes smooth muscle and so may interfere with oesophageal motility

   ☐ D   You suggest she sees a psychologist

   ☐ E   You wonder about CREST syndrome and so arrange oesophageal physiology studies

2.22 **A pharmaceutical company approaches you for ideas on novel methods for fighting obesity. You observe that work to identify drugs that may modulate the satiety centre has so far been less successful than work targeted on preventing the digestion and absorption of dietary fat. In considering the mechanism of fat digestion and absorption which one of the following could be possible mechanisms of action for a new anti-obesity drug?**

- ☐ A   Activation of the pancreatic lipase production system
- ☐ B   Chemo-ablation of mucosal endocrine cells
- ☐ C   Encouragement of fatty acid chelation into micelles in the lumen
- ☐ D   Prevention of cholecystokinin release from gastric enterochromaffin cells
- ☐ E   Promotion of the 'ileal brake'

2.23 **A 24-year-old man with ulcerative colitis is concerned that his GP has asked him to take mesalazine as he has found out from the Internet that it may cause infertility. Which one of the following statements is most accurate?**

- ☐ A   Balsalazide offers similar benefits without the side-effects
- ☐ B   He has got his information wrong
- ☐ C   The benefit of remaining in remission from ulcerative colitis (annual reduction in relapse risk from 70% to 30%) outweighs the potential side-effect to which he refers
- ☐ D   The side-effect is unusual and alternatives are no better
- ☐ E   The value of mesalazine in the maintenance of patients with ulcerative colitis as opposed to Crohn's disease is questionable and he need not take the drug

2.24 **A 50-year-old man complains of perspiration, shakiness and difficulty in concentrating, typically lasting a couple of hours after meals. He has recently had definitive surgery for peptic ulcer disease from which he has made an excellent recovery. Of the investigations that may shed light on the matter which one of the following is likely to be the most useful?**

- ☐ A   Empirical trial of tetracycline
- ☐ B   Gastric emptying studies
- ☐ C   Glucose challenge test
- ☐ D   Gut hormone profile
- ☐ E   Hydrogen breath test

2.25 **The local Director of Public Health is investigating a suspected outbreak of food poisoning. Although no organism has been identified, he hopes that by taking a detailed history from each sufferer he may be able to identify the cause and source. Which one of the following statements is true?**

☐ A Bloody diarrhoea that started within six hours suggests *Entamoeba histolytica*

☐ B If contaminated canned foods were the putative source, *Vibrio parahaemolyticus* is suggested

☐ C If only previously fit and healthy individuals were affected, *Escherichia coli* is likely to be the source

☐ D If rice was the putative contaminated food a *Campylobacter* species is likely

☐ E Symptoms of vomiting within four hours and diarrhoea within ten suggest *Bacillus cereus* as a likely cause

2.26 **A 42-year-old man with a 20-year history of poorly controlled ulcerative colitis, involving the whole colon, attends the clinic for a follow-up appointment. Despite taking azathioprine for six months, he reports intermittent rectal bleeding. Investigations show: bilirubin 35 mmol/l, albumin 35 g/l, alkaline phosphatase 400 U/l, alanine transaminase 50 U/l, ANCA +, antimitochondrial antibody –. Which one of the following is the most likely explanation for the abnormal liver function tests?**

☐ A Alcoholic hepatitis

☐ B Idiosyncratic liver damage due to azathioprine

☐ C Metastases from colorectal cancer

☐ D Primary biliary cirrhosis

☐ E Primary sclerosing cholangitis

2.27 A 40-year-old man with Crohn's disease is admitted with weight loss and diarrhoea. On reviewing his symptoms he describes his stools as pale and runny. He recalls colicky abdominal pain and bloating. He is anaemic and his albumin is very low, although his CRP and plasma viscosity were both normal. Which one of the following is the explanation for his symptoms?

- ☐ A   Acquired lactose intolerance
- ☐ B   Active small bowel Crohn's disease
- ☐ C   Bacterial overgrowth secondary to an enterocolic fistula
- ☐ D   Bile salt diarrhoea
- ☐ E   Small bowel strictures

2.28 A 36-year-old woman presented for investigation of infertility. She had scanty periods for three years, but was noted to be anaemic. Her weight had fallen progressively. She also experienced cramp, particularly in the hands. Other than pallor, angular stomatitis and oral aphthous ulcers, there was little to find on examination. Which one of the following is the most likely diagnosis?

- ☐ A   Coeliac disease
- ☐ B   Crohn's disease
- ☐ C   Giardiasis
- ☐ D   Irritable bowel syndrome
- ☐ E   Scleroderma

2.29 After being called to attend a well-man clinic, a 60-year-old male describes a three-year history of 'indigestion' for which he takes antacids. He has taken aspirin 300 mg daily since a myocardial infarction, but continues to smoke 30 cigarettes/day. He has lost a little weight and is clinically anaemic. A barium meal shows a gastric ulcer on the lesser curve. How would you approach the management of this patient?

- ☐ A   Arrange a serological test for *H. pylori* infection and treat if positive
- ☐ B   Arrange a urease breath test and treat if positive
- ☐ C   Co-prescribe a PPI and review his symptoms
- ☐ D   Refer for endoscopy
- ☐ E   Stop the aspirin and review his symptoms

2.30 A 55-year-old man is referred for the investigation of iron deficiency anaemia. He eats a normal diet and has not lost blood from anywhere. There is no family history and no abnormal signs of examination, other than those of anaemia. Proctoscopy is normal. Which one of the following would be your initial investigation in this patient?

- ☐ A   Barium enema
- ☐ B   Barium meal
- ☐ C   Endoscopy
- ☐ D   Red cell scan
- ☐ E   Stool testing for occult bleeding

2.31 A 26-year-old woman presents with a six-month history of colicky lower abdominal pain associated with loose stool. The stool is accompanied by mucus but not blood. Despite urgency she has noted incomplete evacuation and the need to strain during defaecation. Her weight is increasing. During the last 12 months, she has moved house and then lost her job through redundancy. Bearing in mind the most likely diagnosis, what would you do next?

- ☐ A   Arrange a barium enema
- ☐ B   Arrange a colonoscopy
- ☐ C   Reassure her with explanation of the diagnosis, without further investigation
- ☐ D   Refer to a dietitian
- ☐ E   Refer to a debt counsellor

2.32 A 76-year-old man has a PEG (percutaneous endoscopic gastrostomy) tube in place after a stroke. He presents with vomiting (possibly complicated by aspiration) and apparent abdominal pain after being fed by the PEG. Which one of the following is the explanation?

- ☐ A   Brain tumour
- ☐ B   Drug toxicity
- ☐ C   Hiatus hernia
- ☐ D   Migration of the PEG with pyloric obstruction
- ☐ E   Overfeeding

2.33   **A 25-year-old man presents with a history of severe reflux oesophagitis. Which one of the following is the treatment of choice?**

☐   A   Antacids only

☐   B   Antireflux surgery

☐   C H_2-receptor antagonist

☐   D   High-dose PPI, reducing later

☐   E   Prokinetic therapy

2.34   **After being treated for bleeding oesophageal varices, an alcoholic patient with ascites is found to have deteriorating renal function. His creatinine is rising each day and his urine output is falling. How would you treat him?**

☐   A   Continuous ambulatory peritoneal dialysis (CAPD)

☐   B   Dopamine infusion

☐   C   Intravenous saline

☐   D   Paracentesis/albumin/glypressin

☐   E   Spironolactone

2.35   **A 26-year-old woman presents to the Emergency Department with vomiting and drowsiness. She had been unwell for several days. On examination, she has deep jaundice, blood around the lips, sluggish pupils and a decerebrate posture. Which one of the following is the most likely cause of her illness?**

☐   A   Aspirin overdose

☐   B   Hepatitis A

☐   C   Hepatitis C

☐   D   Paracetamol overdose

☐   E   Wilson's disease

2.36 A 46-year-old woman is referred by a dermatologist to whom she presented with generalised itching. She was found to have the following biochemical results: bilirubin 50 mmol/l, alkaline phosphatase 270 U/l, alanine aminotransferase 60 U/l. Which one of the following is the most likely diagnosis?

☐ A   Alcoholic cirrhosis

☐ B   Chronic active hepatitis

☐ C   Haemochromatosis

☐ D   Primary biliary cirrhosis

☐ E   Systemic lupus erythematosus (SLE)

2.37 A 40-year-old alcoholic man presents to the Emergency Department with a history of upper abdominal pain radiating to his back, accompanied by nausea and vomiting. He is shocked and mildly pyrexial. Which one of the following is the most likely diagnosis?

☐ A   Acute cholecystitis

☐ B   Acute pancreatitis

☐ C   Alcoholic hepatitis

☐ D   Opiate withdrawal

☐ E   Perforated duodenal ulcer

2.38 A 36-year-old alcoholic presents with shock due to bleeding oesophageal varices. After resuscitation, which one of the following is the treatment of choice?

☐ A   Intravenous octreotide

☐ B   Intravenous glypressin

☐ C   Oesophageal variceal endoscopic ligation

☐ D   Oesophageal variceal sclerotherapy

☐ E   Transjugular intrahepatic portocaval shunt (TIPS)

.

2.39 A 30-year-old woman with chronic Crohn's disease of the colon is planning to have a child. She has required two to three courses of steroid each year for the last five years. Which one of the following should be offered to her?

☐ A   Azathioprine

☐ B   Continuous oral prednisolone

☐ C   Ciclosporin

☐ D   Infliximab

☐ E   Methotrexate

2.40 A 30-year-old gay man is referred by his GP after liver function tests. The patient presented with a vague flu-like illness, but was noted to be icteric. His LFTs were as follows: bilirubin 50 mmol/l, alkaline phosphatase 90 U/l, alanine aminotransferase 35 U/l. Which one of the following is the most likely diagnosis?

☐ A   Acute hepatitis A

☐ B   Chronic hepatitis B

☐ C   Hepatitis C

☐ D   HIV hepatitis

☐ E   Gilbert's syndrome

2.41 A 70-year-old man presents with dysphagia. For 30 years he has experienced regular episodes of heartburn. An endoscopic biopsy shows Barrett's oesophagus with high-grade dysplasia. Which one of the following would you use in the first instance to treat this patient?

☐ A   Antireflux surgery

☐ B   Laser ablation

☐ C   Oesophagectomy

☐ D   PPI treatment with repeat endoscopy in three to six months

☐ E   Proton pump inhibitor alone

2.42 A 46-year-old woman presents with rectal bleeding. She reports that she has had difficult defaecation for some years and has had to strain to pass her stools, which are hard. The blood she has observed coats or follows her stool, rather than being mixed with it. Sigmoidoscopy reveals a raised ulcerated lesion on the anterior wall of the lower rectum. Which one of the following is the most likely diagnosis?

- ☐ A   Crohn's disease
- ☐ B   Haemorrhoids
- ☐ C   Lymphogranuloma venereum (LGV)
- ☐ D   Rectal carcinoma
- ☐ E   Solitary rectal ulcer

2.43 A 70-year-old former POW with chronic obstructive pulmonary disease (COPD) presents with a two-month history of rectal bleeding and diarrhoea. On examination he has a hyperinflated chest with widespread wheeze. Sigmoidoscopy shows multiple polypoid lesions in the rectum. Which one of the following is the most likely diagnosis?

- ☐ A   Antibiotic diarrhoea
- ☐ B   Familial adenomatous polyposis
- ☐ C   Pneumatosis coli
- ☐ D   Schistosomiasis
- ☐ E   Villous rectal cancer

2.44 A 36-year-old presents with painless rectal bleeding. He is a gay man and has had several sexual relationships in the months prior to his symptoms. There are no signs on physical examination except on sigmoidoscopy, which shows a florid proctitis. Biopsies show inclusion bodies in the mucosa. Which one of the following is the correct diagnosis?

- ☐ A   Cytomegalovirus (CMV) proctitis
- ☐ B   Herpes
- ☐ C   Lymphogranuloma venereum (LGV)
- ☐ D   Solitary rectal ulcer
- ☐ E   Syphilis

2.45   A 20-year-old man presents with massive haematemesis. He drinks little
        alcohol and does not inject drugs. His past medical history is unremarkable
        except for a prolonged stay on SCBU after being born prematurely. His
        spleen is palpable, but he has no stigmata of chronic liver disease. Which
        one of the following is the underlying diagnosis?

☐   A   Cirrhosis secondary to hepatitis C

☐   B   Cryptogenic cirrhosis

☐   C   Lymphoma

☐   D   Portal vein thrombosis

☐   E   Primary biliary cirrhosis

2.46   A 60-year-old Welsh sheep farmer is admitted for routine hip replacement
        surgery. On examination he is noted to have hepatomegaly.
        Ultrasonography reveals multiple cyst lesions with echogenic areas within
        the cysts. Which one of the following is the most likely diagnosis?

☐   A   Haemangioma

☐   B   Hydatid disease

☐   C   Necrotic metastases

☐   D   Polycystic disease

☐   E   Simple hepatic cysts

2.47   A 66-year-old man reports a six-month history of diarrhoea. He has had
        diabetes for ten months. Dietary measures were inadequate, so his GP
        prescribed escalating doses of metformin. Which one of the following is the
        most likely cause of his diarrhoea?

☐   A   Bacterial overgrowth

☐   B   Bile salt diarrhoea

☐   C   Chronic pancreatitis

☐   D   Irritable bowel syndrome due to concerns about ill health

☐   E   Metformin

2.48   One week after a colectomy with ileostomy for Crohn's disease, a 26-year-old woman begins to experience stomal diarrhoea. The pain around her stoma had started to settle, but increased again. Investigations show her CRP to have risen and her albumin to have fallen. Which one of the following is the cause of her problem?

☐   A   Antibiotic diarrhoea

☐   B   Bile salt diarrhoea

☐   C   Functional diarrhoea due to her disquiet about her stoma

☐   D   Recurrent Crohn's disease

☐   E   Peristomal abscess

2.49   A 32-year-old man with dysphagia is found to have a hypertonic lower oesophageal sphincter with no peristalsis in the body of the oesophagus. Which one of the following is the treatment of choice?

☐   A   Antireflux surgery

☐   B   Botulinum toxin injection

☐   C   Heller's myotomy

☐   D   Domperidone

☐   E   PPI therapy

2.50   After eating a very large Sunday lunch, a 42-year-old man vomits several times before experiencing severe chest pain. On presentation to the Emergency Department, he is shocked. His ECG is normal, but his CXR shows some shadowing in the left lower zone. Which one of the following is the diagnosis?

☐   A   Boerhaave's syndrome

☐   B   Gastritis

☐   C   Mallory–Weiss tear

☐   D   Myocardial infarction

☐   E   Oesophagitis

NEPHROLOGY

Best of Five

Questions

NEPHROLOGY: 'BEST OF FIVE' QUESTIONS

For each of the questions select the ONE most appropriate answer from the options provided.

3.1 **A comatose 18-year-old girl has acute renal failure two days after taking a multiple drug overdose. For the removal of which drug is haemodialysis most likely to be effective?**

☐ A Amiodarone

☐ B Digoxin

☐ C Lithium

☐ D Paraquat

☐ E Phenytoin

3.2 **An 84-year-old hypertensive lady presents with renal failure requiring dialysis. Which one of the following features is most useful in distinguishing between an acute and chronic cause of her renal failure?**

☐ A Haemoglobin level of 11.6 g/dl

☐ B Kidney sizes of 6 cm and 5 cm on ultrasound

☐ C Left ventricular hypertrophy (LVH) on ECG

☐ D Parathyroid hormone level of 7.9 pmol/l

☐ E Phosphate of 2.39 mmol/l

3.3 **You are asked to see a 41-year-old alcoholic patient who has established hepatorenal syndrome. He is hypotensive, oliguric and has evidence of early encephalopathy. Which one of the following therapeutic measures is most likely to improve his prognosis?**

☐ A Haemodialysis

☐ B Liver transplantation

☐ C Plasma expansion with colloid to achieve a central venous pressure (CVP) reading of 8–10 cm

☐ D Promoting a diuresis with furosemide (frusemide)

☐ E Renal transplantation

3.4 **In a 45-year-old man with acute renal failure which one of the following is most likely to be correct?**

☐ A Hypocomplementaemia suggests an autoimmune causation

☐ B In oliguria, dopamine should be used to promote a diuresis

☐ C Low plasma sodium reflects salt-wasting in the renal tubule

☐ D Non-oliguria carries a better prognosis for long-term renal function than oliguria

☐ E Obstruction is excluded by polyuria

3.5 **Which one of the following statements most accurately describes function of a normal kidney?**

☐ A Ammonium excretion in the urine is greater in a chronic than in an acute metabolic acidosis

☐ B Distal secretion of potassium is decreased by acetazolamide

☐ C Increased parathyroid hormone increases tubular reabsorption of phosphate

☐ D Metabolic alkalosis leads to decreased secretion of potassium

☐ E Tubular reabsorption of phosphate does not decrease with increased dietary phosphate intake

3.6 **In which one of the following circumstances is renal excretion of water most likely to be increased?**

☐ A Chronic renal failure

☐ B Early phase of acute tubular necrosis

☐ C Hyperkalaemia

☐ D Hypokalaemia

☐ E Secondary hyperaldosteronism

3.7 **In the kidney, which one of the following statements most accurately describes normal function?**

☐ A Glomerular filtration is favoured if a molecule is negatively charged

☐ B Glomerular filtration is increased by efferent arteriolar constriction

☐ C Glomerular filtration leads to approximately 360 litres of filtrate per day

☐ D Glomerular filtration results from a net filtration pressure of 30 mmHg

☐ E Glomerular filtration results in a filtration fraction of 40%

3.8 **In a woman who is 36 weeks pregnant, which one of the following results is a cause for concern?**

☐ A   Creatinine 85 μmol/l

☐ B   Glomerular filtration rate (GFR) 149 ml/min

☐ C   Magnesium 0.4 mmol/l

☐ D   Urate 0.7 mmol/l

☐ E   Urea 1 mmol/l

3.9 **Which one of the following statements regarding renal clearance is true of a normal-functioning kidney?**

☐ A   Clearance of a substance is the volume of blood cleared of that substance in one minute

☐ B   Clearance of a substance that is neither secreted nor reabsorbed is a measure of renal plasma flow

☐ C   Clearance of inulin is approximately normal when plasma inulin = 0.01 mg/ml, urinary inulin = 0.08 mg/ml and the urinary flow rate = 60 ml/h

☐ D   Clearance of penicillin is increased by probenecid

☐ E   Clearance of urea is an accurate measurement of glomerular filtration rate in the hydrated state

3.10 **In a normal-functioning kidney which one of the following is most likely to increase urinary sodium excretion?**

☐ A   Decrease in GFR of 10%

☐ B   Fall in renal arterial pressure of 15 mmHg

☐ C   Increase in plasma protein concentration

☐ D   Increase in renal sympathetic nervous activity

☐ E   Increase in venous volume

3.11 **A healthy individual has arterial blood gases measured at 10, 000 feet. The arterial P_{CO_2} is low. Which one of the following best represents the renal response to this fall in P_{CO_2}?**

☐ A   Compensation by a rise in pH

☐ B   Compensation predominantly occurring at the proximal tubule

☐ C   Full correction of blood gas measurement of carbon dioxide

☐ D   The renal response leads to a rise in plasma bicarbonate

☐ E   The renal response leads to volume expansion

3.12 **In a healthy individual which one of the following is an accurate statement regarding renin?**

☐ A   Decreased renin release increases thirst

☐ B   Decreased renin release leads indirectly to vasoconstriction

☐ C   Renal cortical ischaemia does not lead to increased renin release

☐ D   Renin release decreases in response to sodium depletion

☐ E   Renal sympathetic nervous stimulation causes increased renin release

3.13 **In a 74-year-old man requiring renal replacement therapy which one of the following factors would best indicate that the patient should commence continuous ambulatory peritoneal dialysis (CAPD) rather than haemodialysis?**

☐ A   BMI of 34 kg/m^2

☐ B   Deforming rheumatoid arthritis

☐ C   Grade III cardiac failure

☐ D   Chronic obstructive pulmonary disease (COPD)

☐ E   Previous multiple abdominal adhesions

3.14 **Which one of the following in a patient with acute renal failure indicates the most urgent need for dialysis?**

☐ A   Asterixis

☐ B   Hiccoughing

☐ C   Hyperkalaemia of 7.0 mmol/l

☐ D   Pericarditis with a pericardial rub

☐ E   Peripheral neuropathy

3.15 **A 40-year-old man is found to be uraemic. Which one of the following facts from the history is most suggestive of a diagnosis of retroperitoneal fibrosis?**

☐ A   He had childhood haematuria

☐ B   He previously worked in an iron foundry

☐ C   He takes atenolol for hypertension

☐ D   He takes paracetamol for fibrositis

☐ E   Three of his children had haemolytic disease of the newborn

3.16   **In a patient with moderate renal failure (GFR 25–50 ml/min) which one of the following is most common?**

☐   A   Childhood growth retardation due to growth hormone deficiency

☐   B   Decrease in GFR as a response to good control of hypertension

☐   C   Hypercalciuria rather than hyperparathyroidism

☐   D   Oliguria rather than polyuria

☐   E   The blood insulin level is disproportionately high for the blood glucose level

3.17   **Which one of the following diagnoses is most likely to be correctly made utilising the renal imaging investigations given?**

☐   A   Dehydration by good quality intravenous urograms

☐   B   Normal renal pathology by measurement of large kidneys on ultrasound

☐   C   Reflux nephropathy by coarse kidney scarring on intravenous urograms

☐   D   Renal obstruction by static radionuclide scanning

☐   E   Retroperitoneal fibrosis by medial ureteric displacement on intravenous urograms

3.18   **A 33-year-old woman presents with nephrotic syndrome and membranous glomerulonephritis is suspected. Which one of the following is most likely to support this diagnosis?**

☐   A   End-stage renal failure occurring within six months of presentation

☐   B   Highly selective proteinuria

☐   C   IgM deposits within the basement membrane

☐   D   Previous presentation with nephritic syndrome

☐   E   The occurrence of renal vein thrombosis

3.19   **Which one of the following statements is the most accurate concerning IgA nephropathy?**

☐   A   Glomerular crescents may occur during episodes of macroscopic haematuria

☐   B   It is an uncommon form of glomerulonephritis

☐   C   Loin pain may occur due to bleeding from peripheral renal arteries

☐   D   Most patients affected will require dialysis treatment

☐   E   The degree of proteinuria does not relate to prognosis

3.20 A 64-year-old man with renal failure develops acute loin pain and haematuria. Doppler ultrasound confirms he has a renal vein thrombosis. Which one of the following is the most likely underlying disease?

- ☐ A   Chronic pyelonephritis
- ☐ B   IgA glomerulonephritis
- ☐ C   Interstitial nephritis
- ☐ D   Reflux nephropathy
- ☐ E   Renal amyloidosis

3.21 Patients with which one of the following inherited diseases are most likely to have a renal tubular defect?

- ☐ A   Childhood polycystic kidney disease
- ☐ B   Cystinosis
- ☐ C   Noonan's syndrome
- ☐ D   Vesico-ureteric reflux
- ☐ E   von Hippel–Lindau syndrome

3.22 A 55-year-old woman presents with renal failure. Which one of the following features is most consistent with a diagnosis of vesico-ureteric reflux?

- ☐ A   Age at presentation
- ☐ B   Normal DMSA (dimercaptosuccinic acid) scan
- ☐ C   Normal micturating cystourethrography
- ☐ D   Positive anti-neutrophil cytoplasmic antibody (ANCA)
- ☐ E   Presentation with acute renal failure

3.23 In an Asian man with active tuberculosis of the urinary tract which one of the following is most likely to occur?

- ☐ A   Microscopic haematuria
- ☐ B   Night sweats
- ☐ C   Normal chest X-ray
- ☐ D   Persistent pyuria
- ☐ E   Raised serum angiotensin-converting enzyme (ACE) levels

3.24 **In patients with distal (type 1) renal tubular acidosis which one of the following statements is correct?**

☐ A A raised creatinine level is a cardinal feature

☐ B Hypokalaemia is not a common feature

☐ C The disease is not inherited

☐ D Renal calculi occur in less than 50% of patients

☐ E There is reduced ammonia formation despite a normal GFR

3.25 **In a patient who is approaching end-stage renal failure which one of the following drugs is the safest to use?**

☐ A Ibuprofen

☐ B Lisinopril

☐ C Mesalazine

☐ D Omeprazole

☐ E Oxytetracyline

3.26 **Which one of the following is true with regard to cholesterol embolisation?**

☐ A It is a rare cause of renal damage

☐ B It is best diagnosed by arteriography

☐ C It is often associated with blue mottling of the hands

☐ D It is usually manifest by loin pain and frank haematuria

☐ E It is often associated with eosinophilia

3.27 **Which one of the following is true of hepatitis C infection with regard to the kidney?**

☐ A Membranous glomerulonephritis is typical

☐ B Pulsed methylprednisolone may be used in treatment

☐ C Renal remission is rare

☐ D The disease is mediated by cold agglutinins

☐ E There is direct viral infection of the glomerular endothelium

3.28 **Which one of the following is typical of a renal biopsy in a patient with diabetic nephropathy?**

☐ A Diffuse glomerular capillary thickening and basement membrane spikes

☐ B Green birefringence on staining with Congo red

☐ C Intracapillary hyaline thrombi

☐ D Mesangial hypercellularity and fibrinoid necrosis

☐ E Mesangial widening, basement membrane thickening and capillary obliteration

3.29 **Which one of the following is characteristic of vitamin D-resistant rickets?**

☐ A Elevated 1,25-dihydroxycholecalciferol

☐ B Expression confined to males

☐ C Glycosuria

☐ D Impaired phosphate excretion

☐ E Normal parathyroid hormone levels

3.30 **Which one of the following is true of the complications of renal transplantation?**

☐ A CMV matching of donor and recipient is essential

☐ B Gastric ulceration is partly attributable to increased rate of *Helicobacter pylori* carriage

☐ C *Pneumocystis* infection typically occurs at around one year post-transplant

☐ D Reverse barrier nursing for ten days after surgery is mandatory

☐ E The major cause of mortality is malignancy

3.31 **Which one of the following is true for most patients with moderate chronic renal impairment?**

☐ A Alcohol is contraindicated

☐ B Dairy products are a useful source of calcium

☐ C Fluid intake should be 2–3 litres per day

☐ D The diet should be high in cholesterol

☐ E Very low protein diet is beneficial

3.32   In the treatment of poisoning which one of the following is true?

- ☐ A   Haemodialysis following death cap mushroom ingestion does not affect mortality despite good toxin removal
- ☐ B   Haemodialysis is ineffective for salicylate poisoning if coma and acute renal failure have ensued
- ☐ C   Haemodialysis is useful for amitriptyline poisoning
- ☐ D   Peritoneal dialysis is generally preferable to haemodialysis
- ☐ E   Use of bicarbonate as a dialysate buffer is contraindicated

3.33   Which one of the following is true of renal involvement in HIV infection?

- ☐ A   Antiviral therapy is of little benefit in HIV-associated nephropathy
- ☐ B   HIV-associated nephropathy is indistinguishable histologically from focal segmental glomerulosclerosis
- ☐ C   HIV-associated nephropathy typically presents with nephrotic-range proteinuria
- ☐ D   Hypernatraemia is common in HIV infection
- ☐ E   Renal involvement is common in AIDS

3.34   Which one of the following is therapeutically useful in cystinuria?

- ☐ A   Allopurinol
- ☐ B   Cysteamine
- ☐ C   Desferrioxamine
- ☐ D   Penicillamine
- ☐ E   Potassium citrate

3.35   Which one of the following is not used in the treatment of renal stone disease?

- ☐ A   Bendroflumethiazide (bendrofluazide)
- ☐ B   Cholestyramine
- ☐ C   Ibuprofen
- ☐ D   Prednisolone
- ☐ E   Pyridoxine

3.36 A 24-year-old known epileptic is admitted to the Emergency Department in status epilepticus. He is treated with intravenous phenytoin. Some 48 hours later he is found to have acute renal failure. Blood results are as follows: potassium 7.1 mmol/l, creatinine 782 μmol/l, corrected calcium 1.9 mmol/l, phosphate 3.1 mmol/l. What simple procedure would be most useful diagnostically?

- ☐ A BM stix
- ☐ B Electrocardiogram
- ☐ C Fundoscopy
- ☐ D Plain abdominal X-ray
- ☐ E Dipstick urinalysis and microscopy

3.37 Which one of the following is not typically associated with reduced serum complement activity?

- ☐ A Acute post-streptococcal nephritis
- ☐ B Anti-glomerular basement membrane disease
- ☐ C Essential mixed cryoglobulinaemia
- ☐ D Lupus nephritis
- ☐ E Type II mesangiocapillary glomerulonephritis

3.38 Which one of the following examination findings in a patient with renal disease is likely to be helpful in determining the aetiology of the condition described?

- ☐ A Adenoma sebaceum in a patient with microscopic haematuria
- ☐ B Grade 2 hypertensive retinopathy in a patient presenting with creatinine of 647 μmol/l
- ☐ C Hot, tender, swollen leg in a patient with proteinuria of 7 g/24 h
- ☐ D Partial lipodystrophy in a patient with a creatinine of 150 μmol/l and normal urinary sediment
- ☐ E Truncal obesity, thin skin and striae in a patient with a creatinine of 270 μmol/l and proteinuria of 1.5 g/24 h

3.39 **Which one of the following features would make a diagnosis of post-streptococcal glomerulonephritis unlikely?**

- [ ] A Infection two weeks ago with an α-haemolytic streptococcus
- [ ] B Patient is a seven-year-old girl
- [ ] C Proteinuria of 1.1 g/24 h
- [ ] D No elevation of antistreptolysin titre
- [ ] E No impairment of renal function at presentation

3.40 **Which one of the following is true with regard to blood pressure and pregnancy?**

- [ ] A Eclampsia can occur without previous hypertension
- [ ] B It is important to use Korotkoff phase V for blood pressure measurement
- [ ] C The accepted threshold for physiological proteinuria is 0.8 g/24 h
- [ ] D The physiological fall in blood pressure is due to reduced cardiac work
- [ ] E The risk of pre-eclampsia increases with each subsequent pregnancy

3.41 **Which one of the following is true with regard to the management of renal osteodystrophy?**

- [ ] A A high cheese diet is a useful way of increasing calcium intake
- [ ] B Phosphate binders must be taken on an empty stomach
- [ ] C Severe hyperphosphataemia is a contraindication to the administration of 1,25-hydroxy-vitamin D
- [ ] D Surgical removal of severely enlarged glands is often necessary in secondary hyperparathyroidism
- [ ] E The desferrioxamine stimulation test is useful to diagnose iron overload

3.42 **Which one of the following is true with regard to proteinuria?**

- [ ] A Urinary protein excretion of 3 g/l, in conjunction with microscopic haematuria, may be attributable to strenuous exercise
- [ ] B In orthostatic proteinuria, the proteinuria is only present in recumbency
- [ ] C Membranous glomerulonephritis is a major cause of the nephrotic syndrome in young adults
- [ ] D Microalbuminuria is diagnosed by Albustix testing
- [ ] E Pathological proteinuria is pathognomonic of glomerular pathology

3.43 **Which one of the following patients is least likely to develop clinically evident diabetic nephropathy within the next year?**

- ☐ A A 43-year-old man who has had type 1 diabetes mellitus (DM) for 11 years, and who has early retinopathy
- ☐ B A 50-year-old woman with no past medical history, found on routine testing to have glycosuria +++
- ☐ C A 60-year-old man who developed type 1 DM 43 years ago
- ☐ D A Caucasian subject 17 years after development of type 2 DM
- ☐ E A Japanese subject 17 years after development of type 2 DM

3.44 **Which one of the following is not a common feature of the acute phase of haemolytic uraemic syndrome (HUS)?**

- ☐ A Hypercalcaemia
- ☐ B Hyponatraemia
- ☐ C Neutrophilia
- ☐ D Reticulocytosis
- ☐ E Thrombocytopenia

3.45 **Which one of the following is not a contraindication to peritoneal dialysis?**

- ☐ A Acute renal failure in childhood
- ☐ B Chronic obstructive pulmonary disease
- ☐ C Recent surgery for abdominal aortic aneurysm
- ☐ D Salicylate poisoning
- ☐ E Severe malnutrition

3.46 **In a healthy man, on a normal diet of 70 g protein and 4 g sodium each day, which one of the following is untrue?**

- ☐ A The minimum required water intake is approximately 1.35 l/day
- ☐ B The net insensible water loss is approximately 0.2 l/day
- ☐ C The obligated urine volume is approximately 0.8 l/day
- ☐ D Water intake of ten litres in one day would not result in hyponatraemia
- ☐ E Water loss in stools is less than 0.05 l/day

3.47   **Which one of the following is the most important cause of death among UK patients with end-stage renal failure (ESRF)?**

☐ A   Cardiac/vascular

☐ B   Complications of transplantation

☐ C   Infection

☐ D   Malignancy

☐ E   Voluntary withdrawal of dialysis/suicide

3.48   **Which one of the following statements concerning haematuria is untrue?**

☐ A   A high proportion of distorted red cells suggests a glomerular origin

☐ B   Family history may be relevant

☐ C   Haematuria is visible at a concentration of approximately 5 ml blood per litre of urine

☐ D   Haematuria rarely results from standard warfarinisation in the absence of structural lesions

☐ E   1 g/day of proteinuria would be expected with haematuria due to a bladder malignancy

3.49   **Which one of the following is likely to be therapeutically useful in a patient suffering from hepatorenal syndrome?**

☐ A   Angiotensin-converting enzyme (ACE) inhibition

☐ B   Combined liver and kidney transplantation

☐ C   Continuous veno-venous haemofiltration

☐ D   Correction of hyponatraemia with normal saline infusion

☐ E   Volume expansion with colloid

3.50   **In the investigation of a neonate with renal cysts, which one of the following is most likely to allow differentiation between autosomal recessive and autosomal dominant polycystic disease?**

☐ A   Intravenous pyelogram (IVP) of patient

☐ B   Liver ultrasonography of patient

☐ C   Renal biopsy of patient

☐ D   Renal ultrasonography of patient

☐ E   Renal ultrasonography of teenage parents

ENDOCRINOLOGY: 'BEST OF FIVE' ANSWERS

1.1   A: He is being treated for diabetes insipidus

Craniopharyngiomas are often cystic and arise from embryonic remnants of Rathke's pouch above the pituitary. As a result, they frequently cause hypothalamic damage and associated diabetes insipidus as well as visual field defects, but infrequently cause hypopituitarism. They are not particularly radiosensitive, do not respond to bromocriptine, and the mainstay of treatment is surgical debulking or cyst drainage, which may have to be performed more than once. In contrast, true pituitary tumours, if large, frequently cause hypopituitarism but rarely cause diabetes insipidus (although this may follow surgical intervention) as this requires damage to the hypothalamus.

1.2   C: It is found at low levels in starvation

Insulin-like growth factor 1 (IGF-1) is synthesised by the liver in response to growth hormone (GH) from the pituitary and mediates most of the actions of GH. Levels are high in acromegaly and measuring levels in this condition may be of some diagnostic use. Levels fall within 24 hours of starvation. At least six specific binding proteins for insulin-like growth factor exist and cleavage of them is an important regulatory step in the action of IGF-1. Circulating levels are very much greater than insulin but there is relatively little cross-talk at the insulin receptor until levels are extremely high.

1.3   A: Arginine

GH release is stimulated by stress, hypoglycaemia, amino acids (especially arginine), growth hormone releasing hormone (GHRH) and the hexapeptide related to the metenkephalins. It is inhibited by somatostatin (octreotide) and glucose. Standard tests of GH release include the insulin-hypoglycaemia stress test and GHRH-arginine stimulation. GH secretion is greater during sleep but this is not an easily reproducible test.

1.4   A: Adrenal replacement therapy should be started before thyroxine

In hypopituitarism, GH and gonadotrophin production are lost early. It is now appreciated that many patients benefit from GH replacement for improved mood, lipid profile, muscle strength and bone density. Testosterone therapy restores potency and libido but not fertility. It requires injections of follicle stimulating hormone (FSH) and HCG (to replace LH) and is used for around six months until semen can be stored. It is essential that adrenal replacement is given before thyroxine as unopposed thyroxine may accelerate metabolism of the remaining cortisol, thereby precipitating an addisonian crisis. Renin and aldosterone continue to be secreted in hypopituitarism and hence mineralocorticoid replacement is rarely required.

1.5   B: A pituitary tumour can usually be seen on MRI scanning

In the vast majority of cases, acromegaly is caused by a pituitary tumour and this is easily visible on MRI scanning (in contrast to tumours causing Cushing's syndrome for example). Prolactin is often co-secreted and moderately raised levels may be present. Diagnosis is made by failure to suppress growth hormone levels during a glucose tolerance test and a raised IGF-1 level is usually present. Treatment reduces sweating and some soft tissue swelling, but the majority of the acromegalic features do not resolve. An increase in both colonic polyps (adenomatous, pre-malignant) and colon cancer is reported and routine colonscopy of patients with active disease is often recommended.

1.6   D: It is synthesised in the hypothalamus

ADH (vasopressin) is synthesised in the hypothalamus and transported via axons to the posterior pituitary. It is a cyclic nonapeptide which, although it is stored bound to neurophysin, circulates in the blood mostly in the unbound form. Its release is promoted by carbamezapine (resulting in 'inappropriate ADH syndrome') and is suppressed by alcohol.

1.7   D: Lithium therapy

Failure of secretion of ADH results in cranial DI whereas tubular resistance to ADH action underlies the nephrogenic form. Untreated, dehydration results in a raised serum sodium, but the condition is not fatal in conscious individuals with access to water, as the thirst mechanism drives the individual to drink as required. Lithium, hypercalcaemia, hypokalaemia and drugs (including demeclocyline) inhibit the action of ADH and result in nephrogenic DI. Nephrogenic DI can be inherited in a sex-linked form and is paradoxically ameliorated to some degree by thiazide diuretics.

1.8   C: Exclusion of treatment with anti-emetic drugs

Galactorrhoea is invariably the result of excess prolactin or increased sensitivity to it. It should not be confused with gynaecomastia in men, which is associated with increased oestrogen action. Gynaecomastia should prompt a search for chronic liver disease, hypogonadism or an oestrogen/HCG-producing occult malignancy of the lung or testis. Raised prolactin levels and galactorrhoea are frequently associated with dopamine-blocking drugs, especially major tranquillisers and anti-emetics, but are rarely associated with antidepressants. If drug side-effects have been excluded, investigation involves thyroid function testing (rarely hypothyroidism induces hyperprolactinaemia via TRH), a prolactin level and imaging of the pituitary. The latter is done because small or moderate elevations of prolactin can be caused by non-functioning and potentially sight-threatening tumours of the pituitary pressing on the pituitary stalk ('disconnection hyperprolactinaemia'). However, the commonest cause in pre-menopausal women is a prolactin microadenoma.

1.9   A: Elevated LH levels

Anorexia is a 'stressed starvation' state with raised cortisol and growth hormone levels but low IGF-1 and a hypothalamic pattern of hypogonadism (low LH, FSH and oestrogen). Secondary amenorrhoea with axillary (but rarely pubic) hair loss is common but presentation earlier in childhood with primary amenorrhoea can occur.

1.10   A: Anosmia

Hypogonadism in a phenotypic male may be due to primary gonadal failure (typically Klinefelter's syndrome, karyotype XXY) with raised gonadotrophins (LH, FSH) or secondary gonadal failure with low LH and FSH. Causes of the latter include delayed puberty, pituitary damage or Kallman's syndrome (isolated LH/FSH failure, often with anosmia). Sex hormone binding levels are raised by oestrogen but reduced by androgen and hence tend to be relatively high in male hypogonadism. Exposure to androgens in utero can cause masculinisation of a female fetus but the result is usually intersex rather than a true phenotypic male.

1.11   D: Radioiodine may not be the ideal first-line treatment

The combination of hyperthyroidism and specific eye signs (other than simply lid retraction and lid lag) strongly suggests a diagnosis of primary hyperthyroidism due to Graves' disease. In this condition the thyroid is stimulated by anti-TSH receptor agonist antibodies and TSH levels themselves are undetectably low. Antithyroid peroxidase antibodies are detectable in up to 90% of cases but these are not believed to be pathogenic. If the woman becomes pregnant, transplacental passage of agonist antibodies (not thyroxine itself, which has a shorter half-life and will be at normal levels after antithyroid drug treatment) can potentially result in neonatal thyrotoxicosis for several weeks although this is rare (around 4% of pregnancies with Graves' disease). In treatment, significant evidence suggests that radioiodine has a greater chance than other treatments of exacerbating the eye disease and should be deferred or given with steroid cover. Restoring euthyroidism rarely improves the eye manifestations and over-treatment (resulting in hypothyroidism) may actually make these worse.

1.12   C: Cardiomyopathy

Profound hypothyroidism is associated with a variety of neurological disturbances, including ataxia, deafness, paranoia, delusions and confusion ('myxoedema madness'). Autoimmune hypothyroidism is associated with an increased incidence of other autoimmune diseases, especially Addison's disease (Schmidt's syndrome) and vitiligo. Multiple serous effusions can occur and cardiac tamponade has been described as well as accelerated coronary artery disease, but cardiomyopathy is not a recognised feature.

1.13   E: Tenderness over the thyroid gland

Thyrotoxicosis due to Graves' disease, toxic multinodular goitre or toxic nodule rarely spontaneously remits. However, destructive thyroiditis due to subacute thyroiditis (also known as post-viral, de Quervain's or granulomatous thyroiditis) spontaneously remits. This is associated with a short history, tenderness over the thyroid gland and a raised erythrocyte sedimentation rate (ESR) (sometimes confused with a viral sore throat), as well as absent uptake of radioiodine. This usually follows a period of transient hypothyroidism. Transient thyroiditis also occurs in the post-partum period and in patients with autoimmune thyroiditis (silent thyroiditis).

1.14   A: Amiodarone therapy

This pattern of thyroid function tests suggests thyrotoxicosis. It is also consistent with over-treatment or factitious ingestion of T4, but not T3 (as the latter would result in a low T4 level). Hyperemesis gravidarum with very high HCG levels can result in mild thyrotoxicosis by cross-reactivity between HCG and TSH at the TSH receptor. Normal pregnancy results in a rise in total T4 but not free T4 and only a slight fall in TSH in the first trimester. Systemic illness results initially in a low T3 followed by a low TSH and in prolonged illness a low T4; a raised free T4 can occur but is unusual. Cytokine therapy (eg interferon-α, interleukin-2) can exacerbate underlying autoimmune thyroiditis and precipitate hypothyroidism. The recovery phase from T cell-depleting therapy (Campath monoclonal antibody treatment) has been associated with Graves' disease but thyrotoxicosis is very rare with cytokine therapy. Amiodarone therapy, however, can produce thyrotoxicosis or hypothyroidism, the former as a result of either iodine overload or a destructive thyroiditis, and can be difficult to treat. Hypothyroidism typically occurs in the first year of beginning amiodarone but thyrotoxicosis can occur at any time.

1.15   C: Persistent generation of cyclic AMP

G proteins are multimolecular complexes that are characterised by their ability to hydrolyse guanosine triphophate (GTP) to guanosine diphosphate (GDP) and are involved in many intracellular processes. In endocrinology they are activated by many membrane receptors (eg the receptors of adrenaline (β), TSH, LH, FSH and GHRH). G proteins themselves activate adenylate cyclase to generate cyclic AMP. In the process of activation, the α-subunit separates from the β- and γ-subunits but it then spontaneously hydrolyses GTP and reforms the α-β-γ trimer. Mutations in the G proteins have been described which prevent this spontaneous inactivation, causing persistent cyclic AMP generation and resulting in tumour formation (eg GH-secreting tumours in acromegaly, but not non-functioning pituitary tumours) or gland overactivity (toxic thyroid nodule, McCune–Albright syndrome). Multiple endocrine neoplasia type II does not involve G proteins. One form of pseudo-hypoparathyroidism is associated with an inactivating G protein mutation but pseudopseudohypoparathyroidism (phenotypic abnormalities of pseudohypo-parathyroidism but normal calcium homeostasis) is not.

1.16   B: An adrenal carcinoma

This lady has Cushing's syndrome, confirmed by the raised 24-hour free cortisols. The short history is suggestive of an aggressive neoplastic process and the strong element of virilisation is suggestive of an adrenal carcinoma. This is further supported by the undetectable ACTH levels as the cortisol from the neoplastic adrenal suppresses the pituitary. The prognosis is very poor in such cases. Cushing's syndrome is most commonly caused by an ACTH-secreting pituitary tumour but in this case, and in the case of ACTH production from a bronchial carcinoid, circulating ACTH levels would be detectable. Squamous cell carcinoma of the bronchus is rarely associated with Cushing's syndrome – the association is with small-cell lung cancer secreting ACTH. In the latter condition, the history is short but the biochemical features predominate (hypokalaemic alkalosis), ACTH levels are high, cushingoid features are typically absent, and extensive lung cancer is readily apparent on chest X-ray.

1.17   C: It causes vasodilatation

Atrial natriuretic peptide, as its name suggests, is a peptide hormone secreted from the myocardium that causes natriuresis (excretion of sodium). It is released under conditions of hypervolaemia (myocardial stretch) and its actions are all consistent with mechanisms to correct the hypervolaemic state: reduced thirst, vasodilatation and excretion of sodium. In the last mechanism it acts directly on the kidney rather than via suppression of aldosterone.

1.18   A: Fatigue

Glucocorticoid deficiency results in rather non-specific fatigue and weakness that responds within hours to glucocorticoid. Postural hypotension may also be a useful indicator but reflects more severe failure, as does hypoglycaemia. Salt craving and hyperkalaemia are manifestations of mineralocorticoid deficiency, which may co-exist.

1.19   A: A female infant will present with intersex

21-Hydroxylase deficiency accounts for around 95% of all congenital adrenal hyperplasia. Homozygous individuals may present with an addisonian crisis (salt-losing in two-thirds of cases) in infancy (with hypotension) and females may present as intersex due to the masculinising effect of excess androgen production from the affected adrenals. Intersex is not likely in boys, but premature puberty may occur. 17-OH progesterone is characteristically very high in this condition as it precedes the enzyme failure in the steroidogenic pathway.

1.20   A: A good response in terms of calcium levels to treatment with calcium and vitamin D

Idiopathic hypoparathyroidism is typically autoimmune in origin. It should be distinguished from pseudohypoparathyroidism which is sometimes associated with short fourth and fifth metacarpals and in which resistance to parathyroid hormone (PTH) occurs, resulting in hypocalcaemia despite raised levels of PTH. Idiopathic hypoparathyroidism is associated with other autoimmune conditions (especially in autoimmune polyglandular failure type 1 where it is associated with mucocutaneous candidiasis, coeliac disease, and adrenal failure), but rarely with hyperthyroidism. It does respond well in terms of raising calcium levels to treatment with vitamin D and calcium. However, calcium levels should be maintained in the low-normal range to avoid hypercalciuria and renal stones.

1.21   C: Serum alkaline phosphatase reflects disease activity

Paget's disease is predominantly a disorder of disordered bone turnover. Serum alkaline phosphatase is raised in more extensive cases and is a useful indicator of active disease and response to treatment. Standard treatment is with bisphosphonates – there is no place for treatment with vitamin D analogues. The disease is often asymptomatic and non-progressive. Indications for treatment include pain, impingement on joints, very high alkaline phosphatase (extensive disease), pressure effects (eg deafness) and high-output cardiac failure.

1.22   B: Hyperparathyroidism

MEN type 1 is associated with mutations in the gene *menin* and results in familial hyperparathyroidism, pituitary tumours and gastrointestinal (GI) neuroendocrine tumours (especially gastrinoma and insulinoma). The major morbidity comes from the GI tumours. There is also an increased incidence of carcinoid. MEN type 2 is associated with mutations in the *RET* proto-oncogene and results in hyperparathyrodism in association with medullary thyroid cancer and phaeochromocytoma. Both of the latter are potentially lethal.

1.23   A: A sulphonylurea screen

Spontaneous hypoglycaemia (not due to over-treatment of diabetes) should always be investigated. Serum insulin levels at the time of hypoglycaemia provide the most important information but C-peptide levels and a sulphonylurea screen on the same blood sample are also helpful. C-peptide and insulin levels are inappropriately high in insulinoma but these results are indistinguishable from occult sulphonylurea abuse. Factitious hypoglycaemia due to occult insulin administration would result in high insulin but not raised C-peptide levels. A glucose tolerance test is of no value in the investigation of fasting hypoglycaemia. Thyrotoxicosis is rarely associated with hypoglycaemia. Hypoadrenalism is, but 24-hour urinary free cortisol is a measure of glucocorticoid excess, not deficiency.

1.24   E: Yearly screening with urinary catecholamines in familial disease

Ten per cent of spontaneous phaeochromocytomas are malignant (less in familial disease), but this can only reliably be determined by the presence of local invasion or metastases. Tumour histology is often very dysplastic, even in lesions that subsequently follow a benign course, a feature common to many endocrine tumours. Malignant disease, when it occurs, is difficult to treat and is not radiosensitive. Benign tumours can also be fatal from hypertensive crises and cardiomyopathy, making it important to screen annually for new tumours in patients with familial disease (including MEN 2). Initial treatment is with α-blockade prior to surgery (unopposed β-blockade can result in a hypertensive crisis). There is no association with islet cell tumours.

1.25   C: High gastrin levels area associated with pernicious anaemia

Although vasopressin has vasoconstrictive effects, the analogue DDAVP does not. Vasopressin secretion is increased by carbamazepine and other drugs that result in inappropriate ADH syndrome. Although administration of calcitonin lowers calcium levels, removal of the C-cells that make this hormone – as occurs with total thyroidectomy – does not appear to affect calcium homeostasis. The failure of acid secretion as seen in pernicious anaemia and with H_2- or proton pump blockade does result in hypergastrinaemia. Glucagon levels are raised in diabetic ketoacidosis, but in long-standing disease the glucagon response to hypoglycaemia fails.

1.26 D: Withhold any antithyroid treatment and repeat thyroid function testing in three weeks

Thyrotoxicosis presenting in pregnancy is due either to Graves' disease or cross-reactive activation of the TSH receptor by the very high HCG levels in the first trimester of pregnancy (the two hormones have a common α-subunit). Characteristics of the latter condition are that it is commonly associated with hyperemesis gravidarum, occurs in the first trimester and subsides spontaneously in the subsequent weeks (as the HCG level falls), is biochemically mild, and is more frequently seen with twin or molar pregnancies. A confident diagnosis cannot be made in the absence of Graves' eye disease and a wait-and-see policy is appropriate if the degree of thyrotoxicosis is mild and the patient clinically well. Propylthiouracil may be used and is safe but is often unnecessary. Radio-nucleotide scans are contraindicated in pregnancy and subtotal thyroidectomy is only indicated in Graves' disease with ongoing thyrotoxicosis in patients intolerant of medication. There are no grounds for advising termination except in a molar pregnancy.

1.27 E: Short Synacthen testing followed by immediate treatment with hydrocortisone

External beam radiotherapy continues to cause pituitary damage for 20 years or more after treatment. It is most likely that this man has now developed pan-hypopituitarism with secondary gonadal failure, but also adrenal failure (low sodium and tiredness but the potassium is not raised as mineralocorticoid function is preserved in secondary adrenal failure) and possibly also secondary hypothyroidism (the TSH is often misleadingly normal but T4 or T3 testing shows a very low value). The most dangerous element here is adrenal failure. Insulin stress testing or treatment with thyroxine (which accelerates metabolism of adrenal steroids) may precipitate a fatal hypotensive crisis. Adrenal failure should be assumed. Short Synacthen testing (with synthetic ACTH and cortisol sampling at 0, 30 and 60 minutes) is safe and if immediately available involves minimal delay. Alternatively, a sample for random cortisol could be saved prior to urgent treatment with parenteral hydrocortisone. Thyroxine and testosterone replacement can be commenced later.

1.28   D: Corticosteroids act more slowly because they act by modulating gene transcription

β-agonists like adrenaline act via cell surface 7-transmembrane receptors and once bound to their ligand activate G proteins that in turn activate the enzyme adenylcyclase. The result is rapid (seconds) generation of cyclic AMP which acts as an intracellular second messenger to mediate the actions of the drug/hormone. Corticosteroids are lipid-soluble but their effects are generated slowly because they act by modulating gene transcription and new proteins must either first be synthesised or existing ones be degraded. However, once generated, these changes in intracellular protein result in prolonged action beyond the serum half-life of the hormone.

1.29   C: A high renin level

Renal artery stenosis results in high renin and high aldosterone levels in contrast to Conn's syndrome in which the aldosterone is high but the renin is characteristically suppressed. While the aldosterone level is high in both cases, it will not discriminate between the two conditions.

1.30   E: 24-hour urinary free cortisol

To distinguish Cushing's syndrome from simple obesity, a 24-hour urinary free cortisol or an overnight low-dose (1 mg) dexamethasone suppression test is typically used. There is loss of diurnal variation in cortisol in Cushing's syndrome. This means that the morning cortisol remains high, but a high evening (midnight) value is strongly suggestive of organic disease. Salivary cortisol measurements can be used to assess this but the assay is not routinely available. Serum potassium is low and bicarbonate high in Cushing's syndrome but these features would also be seen in hypertension treated with a diuretic and are not very specific for Cushing's syndrome. ACTH levels may be inappropriately 'normal' in pituitary-dependent Cushing's. Adrenal or pituitary scanning may show abnormalities in Cushing's but, in the absence of a biochemical diagnosis, radiological abnormalities could be due to non-functioning 'incidentalomas' which are relatively common at both sites.

1.31   B: Basal bolus insulin

The DIGAMI study shows that diabetics treated with intravenous insulin for at least the first 24 hours, followed by subcutaneous insulin for at least three months, have significantly lower mortality rates up to 3.4 years later. This is regardless of the form of treatment they were taking prior to the MI. The mechanism of this is unclear but may be related to the reduction in free fatty acids released as part of the stress reaction. He has a degree of heart failure and renal impairment, meaning that metformin is contraindicated because of the risk of lactic acidosis.

1.32   D: To reduce his insulin to maintain relatively high blood sugars (8–15 mmol/l) for at least three months

This individual has hypoglycaemia unawareness. This is relatively common in long-standing diabetics, particularly in individuals who have very tight blood sugar control and have frequent hypoglycaemic episodes. It appears that the recurrent hypos result in a blunting of the adrenaline (and glucagon) response to hypoglycaemia, making it harder for the individual to detect, take evasive action (eating) and avoid further hypos – hence the phrase 'hypos beget hypos'. A relaxation in diabetic control with reduced insulin doses for three months such that all hyopglycaemic episodes are avoided results in a restoration of hypoglycaemia awareness and is the most appropriate advice. While regular blood sugar testing may help, it is not sustainable in the long term and will not in itself restore hypoglycaemia awareness. Eating every two hours may reduce hypoglycaemic episodes but would result in weight gain and would not be the ideal way to manage this problem.

1.33   B: Aggressive management of hypertension

At the stage of microalbuminuria in diabetic nephropathy, glomerular filtration rates are relatively well preserved and serum creatinine is normal. Aggressive hypertension management down to levels as low as 130/80 mmHg has proved to be the best method of delaying decline in renal function and progression to macroalbuminuria. Good glycaemic control is key to preventing the development of nephropathy in the first place but plays a rather minor role in preventing progression from micro- to macroalbuminuria. Likewise, a low protein diet and aggressive lipid lowering can contribute to maintaining renal function but their role is limited. Diuretics are not contraindicated in diabetic nephropathy and can be used to treat hypertension.

1.34   D: Trans-sphenoidal surgery

The best chance of cure of small- to moderate-sized growth-hormone secreting pituitary tumours causing acromegaly is trans-sphenoidal surgery, with cure rates approaching 70% in experienced centres. With larger tumours, complete cure is unlikely, but it is still appropriate to debulk the tumour and follow with radiotherapy. Octreotide therapy is very effective at lowering growth hormone levels by inhibiting growth hormone synthesis and release. However, it is very expensive, has to be given parenterally at least monthly, does not effect a cure or cause much tumour shrinkage and its exact role in therapy remains to be defined. Only 20% of GH-secreting tumours respond to bromocriptine and yttrium implantation has now given way to the safer procedure of external beam radiotherapy via three overlapping fields.

1.35   C: Hydrocortisone 10 mg mane and 5 mg pm, and fludrocortisone 100 μg mane

In primary adrenocortical failure (Addison's disease) both gluco- and mineralo-corticoid (eg fludrocortisone) replacement therapy is essential. The glucocorticoid treatment should be given at the lowest possible doses to avoid long-term hypercortisolaemia. Possible dosing for glucocorticoid replacement alone includes hydrocortisone 10 mg mane/5 mg pm, or 10 mg bd, prednisolone 5 mg or dexamethasone 0.5 mg. Higher doses of any of these drugs, except in an emergency, is detrimental in the long term, with cushingoid side-effects. Dexamethasone has no mineralocorticoid effect and could precipitate an adrenal crisis if given alone.

1.36   C: Prophylactic thyroidectomy and regular screening for phaeochromocytoma

Multiple endocrine neoplasia (MEN) type 2 comprises hypercalcaemia (hyper-parathyroidism) and two potentially fatal conditions: medullary thyroid cancer (MTC) and phaeochromocytoma. By the time MTC is detectable on thyroid imaging it is unlikely to be curable and patients positive on genetic testing are now being advised to have a prophylactic thyroidectomy, typically before the age of ten years. Bilateral adrenalectomy is a more dangerous procedure and may miss extra-adrenal phaeochromocytomas. Hence routine adrenalectomy is not advised but urinary catecholamine secretion should be measured regularly (eg yearly) followed by imaging if the screen proves positive. Pituitary tumours are a feature of MEN type 1, not of MEN type 2.

1.37   A: A benign course is very likely in such cases

Scattered dark (terminal or non-vellus) facial hairs and an escutcheon (hair between the umbilicus and pubic area) are common in women, as is hair on the lower arms and legs. When associated with menstrual irregularity dating from soon after the menarche or early 20s, by far the most common diagnosis is polycystic ovarian syndrome. Normal or slightly raised levels of testosterone are typically present and a benign course with a 'plateau' in hair growth in the mid-20s is to be expected. Hair on the upper back is unusual. Signs of virilisation comprise clitoromegaly, voice deepening, breast atrophy, and male pattern baldness and indicate very marked increases in androgen levels. In such situations and whenever the testosterone level is markedly raised (eg > 5 nmol/l), screening for adrenal and ovarian tumours is mandatory. Congenital adrenal hyperplasia is also a cause but is usually diagnosed in childhood.

1.38   A: He could be started on a sulphonylurea, taught to test his own capillary glucose levels and be reassessed in one month

This gentleman is relatively thin and young and is likely to have type 1 diabetes. He will have some residual β cell function (insulin production) and in older individuals this may persist for several months or years. Weight loss at presentation is strongly suggestive of type 1 diabetes but does not always occur in this older age group. Urgent hospital admission is not necessary, as he is not ketotic or obviously unwell. However, he should be observed closely as his β cell function may decline rapidly. Metformin is not appropriate. Treatment with a sulphonylurea to augment insulin production seems reasonable in this case but the patient should be reviewed as soon as possible (eg in one month) in case it is proving ineffective or hypoglycaemia has been precipitated.

1.39   A: Amino acids are an increasingly important source of substrates for glucose synthesis

Liver glycogen supplies glucose in the first 12 hours of fasting but is rapidly used up. After this, amino acids are increasingly the source of glucose synthesis, as fatty acids cannot be converted to glucose. Glucagon levels rise within the first 12 hours of starvation and remain high. Mild ketonuria is often detectable in the first 24 hours of starvation as the low insulin levels result in fatty acid mobilisation.

1.40   D: Treatment should commence with a statin

Such a high level of cholesterol in a young person without elevated triglyceride levels strongly suggests heterozygous familial hypercholesterolaemia (LDL receptor defect). This is autosomal dominantly inherited and heterozygotes typically suffer myocardial infarction around the age of 40, consistent with this man's family history. Current treatment is with high doses of HMG-CoA reductase inhibitors. The addition of a fibrate or plasmapheresis is sometimes required. Excess alcohol and uncontrolled diabetes are typically associated with a mixed (raised cholesterol and triglyceride) hyperlipidaemia.

1.41   C: Hyperparathyroidism and malignancy account for 90% of cases

Asymptomatic hypercalcaemia in females in this age group is typically due to hyperparathyroidism. Further investigation, particularly parathyroid hormone estimation, is required to rule out the possibility of malignancy (with bony metastases or parathyroid hormone related protein production). Malignancy and hyperparathyroidism account for 90% of cases of chronic hypercalcaemia. Alkaline phosphatase levels may be raised in both conditions. 'Normal' or raised parathyroid hormone levels in the presence of hypercalcaemia confirm the diagnosis of hyperparathyroidism. In asymptomatic patients with hyperparathyroidism the indications for parathyroidectomy are controversial but include calcium levels above 3.0 mmol/l, hypercalcaemic crisis and renal stones. Calcium levels are usually stable over many years and parathyroidectomy is frequently not required.

1.42   A: It can improve patients' mood

Growth hormone is increasingly being given to adults who have demonstrable deficiency, most commonly due to pituitary tumours. It may raise mood and energy levels, reduce fat and increase lean body mass, prevent osteoporosis and cause favourable lipid changes. Modern therapy is with genetically engineered GH and so carries no risk of CJD. Treatment should be monitored with IGF-1 levels, as the profile of GH itself after injection is unphysiological.

1.43   B: Primary hyperparathyroidism

The hypercalcaemia of primary hyperparathyroidism results in polyuria and polydipsia and can result in renal calculi from the hypercalciuria. It can result in glucose intolerance, whether the calcium is raised or not, and this improves with decreasing the PTH level. Primary hyperparathyroidism is the commonest cause of hypercalcaemia in the community (malignancy is the commonest in the hospital setting).

Schmidt's syndrome is an association of type 1 diabetes, hypothyroidism, hypo-gonadism and Addison's disease. Abdominal pain can be a feature of the presentation of Addison's disease but this disease is associated with hypo-glycaemia, not hyperglycaemia. In a non-diabetic subject severe infection like pyelonephritis can result in hypoglycaemia, not hyperglycaemia. Somato-statinomas are exceedingly rare and are associated with diabetes and steatorrhoea.

1.44   E: Sickle cell screen

Glycation of haemoglobin is a non-enzymatic process that can be artificially lowered where there is increased red cell turnover such as pregnancy, blood loss or haemolysis (thalassaemia and sickle cell anaemia, including their traits). It can be overestimated as high levels of triglycerides or bilirubin can interfere with the assay. Finally it can be difficult to interpret if other compounds bind to the haemoglobin (opiate addiction, uraemia, alcoholism, high-dose aspirin).

1.45   B: Captopril

'Captopril cough' is not infrequent with ACE inhibitors, being present in 7% of patients. It may be more common in women than in men. This side-effect does not occur with the angiotensin II inhibitors, as they do not inhibit bradykinin breakdown. ACE inhibitors have been felt to improve diabetic nephropathy in normotensive patients with type 1 diabetes; this is probably the case although the evidence is not complete. The commonest cause of death is macrovascular complications in type 2 diabetic patients. The important management issue is aggressive control of blood pressure and the agent used is not important.

Beta-blockers can precipitate asthma which can occasionally present with dry cough without wheezing or shortness of breath but this is a less likely answer than captopril. Both doxazosin and nifedipine are usually very well tolerated, though the former can be associated with postural hypotension on initiation of therapy.

1.46   D: Medullary thyroid carcinoma

Medullary thyroid carcinoma (MTC) can secrete a variety of peptides and prostaglandins, resulting in extra-thyroid symptoms. Diarrhoea and sweating are the most common. It is an important tumour to exclude since it can metastasise early and 20-year survival rates following treatment are as low as 44%. Though MTC is usually sporadic, it can be inherited as part of multiple endocrine neoplasia syndrome (MEN). MEN 2A consists of MCT, hyperparathyroidism and phaeochromocytoma, and MEN 2B consists of MCT, phaeochromocytoma and mucosal neuromas. Both types are transmitted in an autosomal dominant fashion.

Acromegaly can also cause sweating, in this case due to sweat gland hypertrophy, but usually not diarrhoea. Cushing's disease also rarely presents with these symptoms. Both these conditions also rarely show such strong family history. Other causes of sweating to remember for the exam are phaeochromocytoma and carcinoid syndrome, which are investigated for by measuring urinary excretion of vanillymandelic acid and 5-hydroxyindoleacetic acid respectively.

1.47   D: Subacute thyroiditis

Subacute thyroiditis classically presents with a painful, tender thyroid gland which feels hard because of the inflammatory infiltrate. There is a phase of thyrotoxicosis with increased secretion of T4 and T3 and a suppressed TSH. It is associated with a raised ESR. Thyroid radioiodine uptake scan shows low uptake due to the inability of the damaged thyroid epithelium to take up iodine. There is then a transitory euthyroid phase which may follow on to a hypothyroid phase. Depending on the amount of damage to the thyroid gland the hypothyroid phase is variable but can last for months and may be permanent (5% of cases). Antithyroid drugs are ineffective and treatment consists of analgesia and, if symptoms are severe, prednisolone.

Biochemical hyperthyroidism followed by hypothyroidism is also seen in post partum thyroiditis though in this case there would be no neck pain and the ESR is normal. They are more likely to be positive for thyroid autoantibodies both before and after presentation, whereas in subacute thyroiditis there tends to be a transient rise in autoantibodies.

1.48   C: Metformin

Metformin is the first choice, as it does not increase appetite like a sulphonylurea. It decreases gluconeogenesis and increases glucose utilisation and improves insulin sensitivity. It is contraindicated in renal or liver failure as it can predispose to lactic acidosis. Phenformin is not licensed in the UK. Acarbose has a lot of gastrointestinal side-effects and poor glucose-lowering effects. Rosiglitazone is a new class of thiazolidinediones licensed in the UK for dual therapy with either a biguanide or sulphonlyurea, ie not on its own and not with insulin.

1.49   D: A moderately raised LH level and a positive withdrawal bleed following Provera challenge

The typical endocrine changes in polycystic ovarian syndrome are a raised LH/FSH ratio with the FSH in the normal range, a normal or mildly raised prolactin, a mildly raised testosterone and a positive (withdrawal bleed present) response to Provera challenge. This last is because although the cycles are anovulatory, the ovary still makes oestrogen in amounts sufficient to prevent osteoporosis and oestrogenise the uterus. High FSH levels are typically seen in primary ovarian failure and a suppressed LH/FSH level with a raised prolactin suggests that hyperprolactinaemia is the primary cause of the amenorrhoea (eg due to a prolactin microadenoma).

1.50   D: Replace gliclazide with basal bolus insulin

There are a few studies using sulphonylureas in pregnancy, but accepted practice presently is to convert all pregnant women with diabetes on oral hypoglycaemic agents to insulin as soon as they are known to be pregnant. Gliclazide can cross the placenta and there is a risk of fetal hypoglycaemia. In addition, diabetic control should be immaculate in order to avoid congenital abnormalities, macrosomia or fetal loss. The best way of achieving this would be with a basal bolus regime with three injections of a short-acting insulin before meals and an intermediate-acting insulin before bed with a snack.

GASTROENTEROLOGY: 'BEST OF FIVE' ANSWERS

2.1   C: Cut the vagus nerve

The vagus nerve is the conductor of the orchestra of acid secretion. A partial gastrectomy will remove the majority of the acid-secreting mucosa. *Helicobacter pylori* causes a relative achlorhydria. High-dose PPIs antagonise the majority of acid-producing proton pumps. Antacids neutralise luminal acid.

2.2   E: Ursodeoxycholic acid will help her symptoms and may delay disease progression

Curiously, steroids are relatively ineffective in modifying disease progression and add to the risk of osteoporosis. Other immunosuppressants, including methotrexate, have been tried but have no mainstream role in disease management. Ursodeoxycholic acid is probably helpful, with some evidence of clinical and biochemical improvement unless already cirrhotic. Serum bilirubin levels remain a useful guide to the timing of transplant despite the use of ursodeoxycholic acid, which may cause the levels to fall. Survival from the onset of symptoms is typically about seven years less than a healthy 74-year-old could normally expect. The cause of the pruritis is unknown.

2.3   E: Start an *N*-acetylcysteine infusion

In any patient in whom a significant paracetamol overdose is suspected it is worth starting an *N*-acetylcysteine infusion pending further information and blood test results. If considered, gastric lavage should be done within four hours of ingestion. Hypoglycaemia may occur in fulminant liver failure. Transplant should be considered if the pH falls below 7.31, the prothrombin time exceeds 100 s or the creatinine exceeds 300 μmol/l. Psychiatric input is helpful in the management of any patient who has taken an intentional overdose, but should only be sought only once the patient is medically stable.

2.4   E: Pernicious anaemia

Pernicious anaemia and chronic pancreatitis may both contribute to vitamin B_{12} deficiency. The latter is unlikely in the absence of a history of alcohol excess or pain. Coeliac disease may present with an anaemia and may be associated with neurological consequences through malabsorption. However, it would normally cause a normocytic or microcytic anaemia as iron absorption is impaired as well as the absorption of folate, and to a much lesser extent than B_{12}. Body stores of B_{12} can last several years without replacement so the relatively short history of weight loss makes poor appetite a much less likely answer. Vitamin C can impair iron absorption.

2.5   D: The use of a non-selective β-blocker such as propanolol to maintain portal pressure below 12 mmHg

Varices found incidentally at endoscopy are termed 'primary'. Those that present with bleeding are secondary. While serial endoscopy and banding, or perhaps less successfully, sclerotherapy, is appropriate for the latter, management of primary varices is more often conservative with the aim to maintain portal pressure below 12 mmHg. Propanolol is the drug most frequently used though some advocate nitrates as an alternative if propanolol is contraindicated. Terlipressin is used to help manage acute bleeding from varices.

2.6   D: It is likely to be at least as cost-effective as screening for cervical cancer

Evidence from ongoing trials in the UK suggests that screening for colorectal cancer, perhaps initially with faecal occult blood testing then flexible sigmoidoscopy for positives, or perhaps with a single flexible sigmoidoscopy for people in the 50–69-year age bracket, could be at least as cost-effective as cervical screening. Colon cancer is common, being the second or third most common cancer in many league tables, but that in itself would not make screening worthwhile were there no readily detectable pre-cancerous phase or no acceptable curative treatment. Rectal cancer is more common in beer drinkers. High consumption of red meat and animal fat is associated with an increased risk of developing colorectal cancer. Curiously the consumption of both has been falling in the UK since the end of World War II. The incidence of colorectal cancer has been falling too.

2.7   E: Troublesome perianal Crohn's disease

HIV infection is often associated with past or present hepatitis B and C infection with which it shares common routes of transmission. Diarrhoea is a troublesome symptom for patients with HIV, sometimes associated with organisms such as *Cryptosporidium* which normally pose no risk for immunocompetent individuals. Although a few case reports suggest that active Crohn's disease may co-exist with advanced HIV infection, more often the immunosuppression due to HIV suppresses Crohn's disease activity.

2.8   B: His GP may have been better advised to refer the patient for oesophagogastroduodenoscopy rather than test for *Helicobacter pylori* serology

Notwithstanding the patient's use of NSAIDs, his symptoms are atypical for peptic ulcer disease in that the pain is central rather than epigastric and his response to PPIs only moderate. In these circumstances, and given his age (over 55 years) the clinician would normally request both upper GI endoscopy and abdominal ultrasound scanning, the latter to look for peptic ulcer disease and cancer, the former for pancreatic disease in particular, especially given a lack of good response to empirical therapy. The *H. pylori* serology does not differentiate between current and past infection. The presence of *H. pylori* in itself does not necessitate its eradication in the absence of peptic ulcer disease, gastritis or gastric cancer, though some patients with non-ulcer dyspepsia, perhaps one in five, will benefit from *H. pylori* eradication treatment. Although colonoscopy could be helpful, the ease and diagnostic options presented by upper GI tract endoscopy would suggest that that should be done first. In any case looser stools may be a class side-effect of PPIs. Trials suggest that *H. pylori* status is not an independent risk factor for development of ulcers in patients on NSAIDs.

2.9   A: A low-alcohol lager

Only the beer contains a proscribed cereal, barley-derived hops.

2.10   C: She must be sent to hospital as she is dehydrated and pyrexial: given the history you are concerned to diagnose and treat any antibiotic-associated complications early

Confusion, pyrexia, dehydration and diarrhoea are all symptoms and signs that may necessitate admission, if only for care, in an elderly person living alone at home – though not every elderly person with just one of these symptoms could be admitted! While metronidazole is the preferred treatment for *Clostridium difficile*-associated diarrhoea in the UK, it too may cause *C. difficile* overgrowth. Relapse after apparently successful treatment is not uncommon.

2.11   A: Her prognosis is better if she abstains from alcohol permanently

The prognosis is related to her smoking, alcohol intake and the presence of cirrhosis. Ten-year mortality is perhaps 30%. Pancreatectomy has a mortality rate that is perhaps as high as 10%. Thirty per cent of patients may have continuing pain afterwards. Resting the pancreas with exogenous pancreatic enzymes may help symptoms though there is little evidence to suggest it improves prognosis.

2.12   C: If she has had her small bowel resected she may be malabsorbing folic acid and so supplementation at a higher than normal dose would be advised

Folic acid supplements are recommended for all pregnant women as their need for folate rises fivefold. Folate is denatured through overcooking. Liver is contra-indicated in pregnancy through concern about its high vitamin A content. Blind loop bacteria tend to consume B_{12} and produce folate.

2.13   C: His family's description of an inversion of his normal sleep pattern

Patients with hepatic encephalopathy may have hyper-reflexia. The pupillary response is maintained. Headache is a rather non-specific symptom. An inability to recall names does not differentiate between causes of impaired cognitive function.

2.14   D: Offer advice on laxatives

Solitary rectal ulcers are typically found on the anterior rectal wall in young women with a history of constipation, and may reflect strain-associated prolapse. While an uncommon cause of anaemia, in this case other more common causes appear to have been excluded. The histology will differentiate between inflammatory bowel disease and solitary rectal ulcer disease but, given the history, a trial of laxatives rather than mesalazine seems an appropriate next step pending biopsy results.

2.15   E: It stimulates pancreatic exocrine secretion

Cholecystokinin is related to secretin. Its actions include causing the gallbladder to contract and stimulating pancreatic production of lipases in response to a fatty meal. While it does delay gastric emptying it does so via a vagal reflex rather than direct action on the muscularis.

2.16   E: The patient has irritable bowel syndrome

The most likely diagnosis is a post-infective irritable bowel syndrome for which his symptoms meet Rome II criteria. They include abdominal pain in the absence of rectal bleeding and weight loss, a variable bowel habit and a feeling of incomplete evacuation, for at least 12 weeks in the last 12 months. Significant overt blood loss is unlikely in the absence of anaemia. Descriptions of odd-shaped stools are common in irritable bowel syndrome. As the final stool emerges from storage in the relatively capacious rectum, stricturing of the colon would be an unlikely cause. Although his postings overseas need to be considered in reaching a diagnosis, common disease remains common. Irritable bowel syndrome may affect up to one in five of the UK population. Chagas' disease causes a destruction of the myenteric plexus and presents with a dysphagia akin to achalasia as well as cardiomyopathy. It would be highly unlikely for a diplomat to contract this disease, which is seen almost exclusively in rural areas of Brazil.

2.17   E: Treatment with penicillamine and zinc should be started

The incidence of Wilson's disease is said to be higher in Japan than elsewhere. Kayser–Fleischer rings are present in the vast majority of patients with neurological manifestations, of which psychiatric illness may be a part. A decision to transplant is made on the basis of a prognostic index that considers bilirubin, transaminase and prothrombin levels. It may not be appropriate in the presence of significant co-morbidity. Ahead of transplant, chelation is the mainstay of therapy.

2.18   B: Most of the bilirubin is likely to be bound to albumin

The likely diagnosis is Gilbert's syndrome whose prevalence is below 10% worldwide and is due to several genetic faults whose common theme is a relative paucity of liver conjugating capacity. It is more common in men than women. A differential could include haemolysis: in a Cypriot this could be due to a thalassaemia trait though in that case the MCV is more likely to be low. Bilirubin (and most substances without more specific carrier proteins) circulates bound to albumin. It would be unusual for primary biliary cirrhosis to present with a raised bilirubin alone. Gilbert's syndrome is a benign condition that requires no monitoring.

2.19   D: Send blood for genetic studies looking for mutations of the *HFE* gene

The diagnosis of haemochromatosis is reliably confirmed on the basis of mutations of the *HFE* gene on chromosome 6. Slowly progressive, there is no absolute urgency in starting treatment before a firm diagnosis has been made. The blood is healthy. Indeed, by being a regular blood donor, a patient with haemochromatosis can postpone the development of phenotypic disease for years. Family members should be screened at leisure.

2.20   B: Endoscopy is needed to rule out other disease

The concern in patients with symptoms of chronic reflux, a common problem among pregnant women and the overweight as well as athletes, is the potential for metaplasia of the lower oesophageal epithelium, Barrett's change. For that reason endoscopy is suggested as the most appropriate investigation in patients with persistent reflux symptoms. Endoscopy may also demonstrate oesophagitis though patients may suffer from reflux symptoms in the absence of overt oesophagitis. In such cases oesophageal pH studies may be helpful though a good response to antacids or PPIs suggests acid-related symptoms.

2.21   B: You arrange upper GI tract endoscopy

Dysphagia (difficulty in swallowing) and odynophagia (painful swallowing) together require investigation unless they settle rapidly with empirical measures. Trials show that a negative endoscopy may in itself in itself help patients' symptoms to settle. Endoscopy is usually done as a precursor to oesophageal physiology studies though barium fluoroscopy may provide information on both structure and motility. Psychological support may be helpful in the management of functional GI disturbance.

2.22   B: Chemo-ablation of mucosal endocrine cells

Activating lipase production and promoting micelle formation and the 'ileal brake', a mechanism whereby peristalsis is inhibited should a fatty load enter the ileum, would all aid fat digestion and absorption. Theoretically, ablation of mucosal endocrine cells that secrete cholecystokinin and secretin *inter alia* could reduce pancreatic exocrine function and the effectiveness of gallbladder contraction in response to a fatty meal and so it should help to relieve symptoms. Cholecystokinin is not released from the stomach.

2.23   B: He has got his information wrong

Sulfasalazine causes a reversible oligospermia. Mesalazine compounds are useful alternatives and are of similar effectiveness in reducing relapse rates in ulcerative colitis. Their role in Crohn's maintenance is less clear.

2.24   C: Glucose challenge test

Dumping syndrome is described. It is due to the rapid delivery of a high glucose load to the small bowel, consequent rapid glucose absorption, hyperinsulinaemia and subsequent hypoglycaemia. Symptoms are best mimicked by administration of a glucose challenge. The other tests, while helpful, tend to be more cumbersome and provide less direct evidence. Gastric emptying studies, for instance with a radioisotope-labelled test meal, may show rapid emptying. A hydrogen breath test will show an early peak as the test meal reaches colonic bacteria more rapidly than normal. Any abnormality in GI hormone levels is likely to be transient. Bacterial overgrowth plays no role in this condition.

2.25   E: Symptoms of vomiting within four hours and diarrhoea within ten suggest *Bacillus cereus* as a likely cause

E. histolytica tends to cause a sudden onset of bloody diarrhoea 12–24 hours after ingestion. *Campylobacter* species are most commonly found in contaminated animal products. Canned foods classically harbour *Clostridium botulinum* toxin. *Vibrio parahaemolyticus* is found in seafood. Enterotoxic *Escherichia coli* can affect young and old, fit and disabled alike, although is more likely to be life-threatening in the very young or frail elderly.

2.26   E: Primary sclerosing cholangitis

This cholestatic picture is due to primary sclerosing cholangitis (PSC). PSC in ulcerative colitis is associated with ANCA in 80% of patients. It is more common in men than in women. Primary biliary cirrhosis is very uncommon in men. Alcoholic hepatitis gives a hepatitic picture, not one of cholestasis. Azathioprine can cause abnormal LFTs, but this usually settles within the first month. Liver metastases are a possibility, but less likely than PSC.

2.27   C: Bacterial overgrowth secondary to an enterocolic fistula

This is a picture of malabsorption for which the main differential diagnoses are active small bowel Crohn's disease and a fistula, with bacterial overgrowth. The laboratory tests do not indicate an inflammatory process. Acquired lactose intolerance can give bloating and diarrhoea, but not anaemia or low albumin. Bile salt diarrhoea is watery, but not associated with colic or systemic symptoms. Strictures are associated with colic, but will not cause anaemia and a low albumin unless there is bacteria overgrowth too. So, only a fistula with overgrowth will fully explain the symptoms.

2.28   A: Coeliac disease

This is a picture of malabsorption. 'Silent' malabsorption of this type strongly suggests coeliac disease. The mouth ulcers are associated with coeliac disease or Crohn's disease but there are no other symptoms to suggest Crohn's disease. In general, giardiasis and Crohn's disease are associated with gastrointestinal symptoms in addition to malabsorption. Scleroderma has characteristic extra-intestinal signs.

2.29   D: Refer for endoscopy

Gastric ulcers, particularly in patients with 'alarm symptoms', should be biopsied. Weight loss and anaemia are alarm symptoms. Benign ulcers rarely if ever present with anaemia. If this patient is found to have a benign ulcer, then his colon should be investigated.

2.30   A: Barium enema

Occult blood loss in a man of this age is due to a caecal cancer until proved otherwise. This is the age at which the incidence of such cancers rises significantly. FOB testing is pointless and, in the absence of overt blood loss, a non-vegetarian either has malabsorption or GI bleeding; a negative FOB would not rule out bleeding. A red cell scan is only useful during an episode of bleeding. Upper GI malignancy is less common, but should be sought if the barium enema is normal.

2.31   C: Reassure her with explanation of the diagnosis, without further investigation

Her symptoms are those of irritable bowel syndrome. In most patients the cause is stress. Investigations are not called for in patients of this age, if at any age. Reassurance with a careful explanation of the problem is all that is usually required.

2.32   D: Migration of the PEG with pyloric obstruction

This is a picture of upper GI obstruction. PEG migration is the most likely diagnosis.

2.33   D: High-dose PPI, reducing later

NICE guidelines support the stance of most gastroenterologists – to use an effective proton pump inhibitor (PPI), the dose of which is reduced once symptoms come under control. In patients of this age, who are unlikely to be taking other drugs and so are not at risk of drug interactions, price is the main determinant of the choice of PPI. A cost-effectiveness study has shown that antireflux surgery is not useful in most patients as they relapse later and then need to take PPI therapy once more.

2.34   D: Paracentesis/albumin/glypressin

This is type 1 hepatorenal failure. It occurs in patients with cirrhosis complicated by ascites and mild stable renal impairment (type 2 hepatorenal syndrome) who then have reduced renal perfusion due to sepsis or blood loss. The untreated mortality is 90% at two weeks, but the paracentesis/albumin/glypressin regimen lowers mortality and corrects renal failure in most patients.

2.35   B: Hepatitis A

The picture is one of fulminant hepatic failure (FHF). Paracetamol and hepatitis A are the most likely causes but the duration of the antecedent history and the absence of a history of paracetamol overdose make hepatitis A the most likely diagnosis. All patients in this condition should be referred to a liver unit. Hepatitis A serology may be negative at presentation.

2.36   D: Primary biliary cirrhosis

Primary biliary cirrhosis (PBC) is the most likely diagnosis. Itching is often the first symptom. PBC is most common in middle-aged women. The LFTs typically show a cholestatic pattern. Antimitochrondrial antibodies are expected.

2.37   B: Acute pancreatitis

This is acute pancreatitis. However, all the others are reasonable differential diagnoses. Opiate withdrawal is not usually accompanied by shock, nor are cholecystitis and alcoholic hepatitis. Fever is present in alcoholic hepatitis, cholecystitis and sometimes in a perforated duodenal ulcer. However, in none of these does the pain usually radiate to the back.

2.38   C: Oesophageal variceal endoscopic ligation

Ligation is the treatment of choice, if an appropriately skilled endoscopist is available. Sclerotherapy is probably the next best choice although glypressin is very useful. TIPS should be reserved as a salvage technique when other approaches have failed.

2.39   A: Azathioprine

Azathioprine is the only option to consider at this stage. Long-term steroids are not indicated in Crohn's disease. Ciclosporin does not work. Infliximab is only licensed for active disease that is refractory to steroids and first-line immunosuppressives. Methotrexate causes miscarriage.

2.40   E: Gilbert's syndrome

The most likely diagnosis is Gilbert's syndrome. The only biochemical abnormality is of the bilirubin. The other diagnoses each show an elevated transaminase when the bilirubin is raised. Gilbert's syndrome is common, although the jaundice is usually only clinically apparent during an intercurrent illness.

2.41   D: PPI treatment with repeat endoscopy in three to six months

There is a significant risk of Barrett's oesophagus and adenocarcinoma arising in such a patient. Peptic strictures may also occur. Severe oesophagitis may lead to dysphagia even without a stricture. Severe dysplasia should be confirmed by repeat endoscopy in the presence of acid blockade. If confirmed, oesophagectomy should be performed.

2.42   E: Solitary rectal ulcer

The site of the lesion is characteristic. Solitary rectal ulcers are associated with straining at stool and trauma (due to digitally assisted evacuation for example). The lesion may resemble a tumour, so a biopsy is essential.

2.43   C: Pneumatosis coli

The gas-filled blebs are characteristic. Pneumatosis coli is associated with COPD and usually presents with rectal bleeding and diarrhoea. Antibiotic diarrhoea may be accompanied by blood and is a reasonable thought in a patient likely to have been exposed to antibiotics, but the duration of the symptoms is too long. The patient is too old to have familial adenomatous polyposis.

2.44   A: Cytomegalovirus (CMV) proctitis

CMV proctitis is painless, unlike herpes proctitis. Inclusion bodies are characteristic.

2.45   D: Portal vein thrombosis

Bleeding oesophageal varices in the absence of signs of chronic liver disease strongly suggest portal vein thrombosis. SCBU treatment is likely to be associated with umbilical vein cannulation with the attendant risk of sepsis and portal vein thrombosis.

2.46   B: Hydatid disease

Hydatid disease is usually asymptomatic. The infestation is acquired by exposure to faeces containing *Echinococcus* eggs. The internal acoustic shadows are the key to the ultrasonographic diagnosis.

2.47   E: Metformin

Metformin is a common cause of diarrhoea. However, all the others are plausible.

2.48   E: Peristomal abscess

Peristomal inflammation will lead to diarrhoea. The investigations are consistent with an abscess. Bile salt diarrhoea only occurs if the colon is in continuity.

2.49   C: Heller's myotomy

The diagnosis is achalasia. Heller's myotomy is the treatment of choice in a young patient. Botulinum toxin is useful for short-term relief of symptoms for patients who are not fit for surgery.

2.50   A: Boerhaave's syndrome

This is a characteristic presentation of this life-threatening disorder. The oesophagus is ruptured during severe vomiting. Perforation usually occurs to the left, giving rise to mediastinal and pericardial emphysema and a left pleural effusion.

NEPHROLOGY: 'BEST OF FIVE' ANSWERS

3.1   C: Lithium

When taken in excessive quantities, many drugs may cause acute renal failure even if this is not the primary symptom. The mechanism is commonly acute tubular necrosis, which may also occur following severe volume depletion. Haemodialysis is poor at removing drugs which have a large volume of distribution (eg amiodarone and paraquat) or are highly protein-bound (eg digoxin and phenytoin). Haemodialysis may still be required to correct metabolic and fluid balance abnormalities that have occurred as a result of the renal failure.

3.2   B: Kidney sizes of 6 cm and 5 cm on ultrasound

The key features suggesting chronicity of renal failure are anaemia (which is usually normocytic), small renal size on ultrasonography, evidence of long-standing hypertension (LVH) and established bone disease. In an elderly patient the presence of LVH would be a less useful indicator than in a patient of younger age, particularly in a hypertensive patient. Hyperparathyrodism is a sign of established bone disease but hyperphosphataemia will often be seen in dialysis-requiring patients even if there is no underlying chronic renal disease.

3.3   B: Liver transplantation

The hepatorenal syndrome results from rescued renal cortical perfusion secondary to the accumulation of vasoactive substances, thought to be either endotoxin or an interleukin, which are normally cleared from the circulation by the liver. Usually oliguria and a daily urinary sodium excretion of < 10 mmol are found. This syndrome has an appalling prognosis. Only dramatic improvement of hepatic function will lead to resolution of the syndrome and hence liver transplantation is the correct answer. Plasma expansion, followed by diuresis promotion and haemodialysis, if necessary, are all correct supportive measures but will not improve long-term prognosis in established hepatorenal syndrome. If the kidneys are transplanted from a patient with hepatorenal syndrome into a recipient with a normal liver they will function normally.

3.4   D: Non-oliguria carries a better prognosis for long-term renal function than oliguria

Dopamine is used in low doses to improve renal blood flow but this does not always lead to a diuresis. It is vital to ensure that a patient with renal failure is adequately hydrated prior to an attempt to stimulate a diuresis. Polyuria may occur in the recovery phase of acute tubular necrosis or as a result of nephrogenic diabetes insipidus, which may itself occur as a result of intermittent or partial obstruction. In all causes of renal failure non-oliguria carries a better prognosis than oliguria. Low plasma sodium almost always implies an excess of body water rather than a true deficit of body sodium: it gives no clue to tubular function. Hypocomplementaemia may occur in the setting of some autoimmune diseases. Rheumatoid vasculitis, systemic lupus erythematosus (SLE) and polyarteritis nodosa are all associated with complement consumption. However, hypo-complementaemia does not imply autoimmune disease and there are many autoimmune conditions (eg anti-neutrophil cytoplasmic antibody (ANCA-) associated vasculitides) in which complement levels are normal.

3.5   A: Ammonium excretion in the urine is greater in a chronic than in an acute metabolic acidosis

Increased ammonium in the urine is part of the kidney's physiological acid–base buffer systems. Ammonium contains an extra hydrogen ion and its excretion is increased as physiological compensation for a metabolic acidosis. Compensation will be greater in a chronic rather than an acute metabolic acidosis. Phosphate homeostasis is directly influenced by dietary intake; an increased dietary intake of phosphate leads to decreased tubular reabsorption of phosphate. PTH causes phosphaturia. In a metabolic alkalosis there are fewer hydrogen ions to 'compete' with potassium ions for tubular exchange with sodium ions, hence a metabolic alkalosis leads to increased potassium secretion. Acetazolamide, a carbonic anhydrase inhibitor, leads to decreased bicarbonate absorption and an increase of distal tubular reabsorption of sodium (sodium and bicarbonate ions combine to increase delivery of sodium ions to the distal tubule). In exchange for sodium ions, there is an increase of potassium secretion brought about by the action of acetazolamide.

3.6   A: Chronic renal failure

In chronic renal failure, nocturia is often an early symptom. This increase of water excretion occurs because of the osmotic diuretic effect of raised urea and increasing insensitivity of the collecting tubules to ADH. Acquired nephrogenic diabetes insipidus is associated with diseases which mainly affect the renal medulla. Hypokalaemic interstitial nephritis and the recovery phase of acute tubular necrosis (ATN) are examples of such diseases. However, hypokalaemia and hyperkalaemia themselves are not commonly associated with increased renal water excretion. Secondary hyperaldosteronism occurs in hepatic and cardiac failure; this state is usually associated with volume overload which occurs in association with a high renin level.

3.7   B: Glomerular filtration is increased by efferent arteriolar constriction

The net filtration pressure is 10 mmHg (hydrostatic pressure – [oncotic pressure + Bowman's capsule pressure]); 45 – (25 + 10) = 10 mmHg. The basement membrane is made up of negatively charged glycoproteins and collagen, so positively charged molecules are favourably filtered. The filtration fraction is GFR/renal plasma flow and is normally 20% ([120 ml per min]/[600 ml per min]). Overall, approximately 180 l/day of filtrate is produced in a normal kidney. An increase of efferent arteriolar constriction is an autoregulatory mechanism to maintain glomerular filtration.

3.8   D: Urate 0.7 mmol/l

In the second and third trimesters of pregnancy GFR increases and this is reflected by a decrease in both urea and creatinine. The serum concentrations of minerals such as magnesium are also characteristically low as a reflection of this. A rising uric acid level is a cause for concern as it is a possible indicator of the onset of pre-eclampsia.

3.9   A: Clearance of a substance is the volume of blood cleared of that substance in one minute

This definition of clearance is correct. GFR is most accurately measured by clearance of a substance that is freely filtered and neither secreted nor reabsorbed (inulin). The formula for clearance of inulin (a polysaccharide which is not a normal constituent of the body) is urinary concentration $\times$ urinary flow rate/plasma concentration, in this case $0.08 \times 60/0.01 = 480$ ml/min; this does not approximate to the normal value of 120 ml/min. Renal plasma flow is measured by clearance of a substance that is both filtered and secreted by the kidney (para-aminohippuric acid; PAH). Even in the hydrated state, 40% of urea is reabsorbed and so urea clearance is not an accurate measurement of GFR. Probenecid reduces tubular penicillin secretion and so reduces penicillin clearance.

3.10   E: Increase in venous volume

Renal sympathetic activity causes an increase in sodium reabsorption and a decrease in urinary sodium excretion. Similarly, a small fall in renal arterial pressure leads to an increase in proximal tubule reabsorption and decreased urinary excretion of sodium. An increase in venous volume leads to baroreceptor (atrial and renal capillary) signals, leading to increased sodium excretion. Increased plasma osmotic pressure increases proximal sodium reabsorption. All these mechanisms are involved in the maintenance of blood volume. Afferent and efferent arteriolar constriction is involved in autoregulation, maintaining GFR and renal blood flow within narrow limits.

3.11   B: Compensation predominantly occurring at the proximal tubule

The renal response to this respiratory alkalosis is compensatory, restoring the pH to normal by metabolic compensation. The response is compensation rather than correction as the fall in the arterial partial pressure of carbon dioxide is not corrected; P_{CO_2} remains low. There is a decrease in the reabsorption of bicarbonate ions which occurs mainly at the proximal tubule. This leads to a further fall in plasma bicarbonate and the pH will fall towards normal. Volume regulation is not a major part of the renal compensatory mechanisms of acid–base disturbances.

3.12   E: Renal sympathetic nervous stimulation causes increased renin release

Renin is a proteolytic enzyme released from the granular cells of the juxta-glomerular apparatus in response to sodium depletion (detected by cells of the macula densa) or volume depletion (detected by atrial and renal capillary baroreceptors). Reduced atrial stretch leads to increased renal sympathetic tone and renin release. Renin acts on angiotensinogen (renal substrate) to produce angiotensin I (later converted to angiotensin II, a potent vasoconstrictor). Angiotensin also stimulates thirst. Redistribution of blood away from the outer renal cortex stimulates renin release which may be relevant to sodium retention in some disease states.

3.13   D: Grade III cardiac failure

A high BMI of 34 implies obesity. Surgical placement of a catheter for CAPD may be technically difficult in obese patients. Another consideration would be the propensity of CAPD patients to become obese through the glucose load of peritoneal dialysis solutions commonly used. CAPD fluid may splint the diaphragm, especially during the night, which makes its use in patients with low respiratory reserve problematic. A patient with previous multiple adhesions may well have recurrent problems which would make CAPD difficult and also give rise to problematic CAPD catheter insertion. Age is not a contraindication to CAPD provided a patient is mentally and physically agile enough to perform CAPD. Severe cardiac failure often leads to cardiovascular instability during haemodialysis sessions and indicates that a patient should commence CAPD in preference to haemodialysis

3.14   D: Pericarditis with a pericardial rub

Pericarditis indicates urgent need for dialysis because of the risk of cardiac tamponade which may occur because of bleeding from the inflamed pericardium. Dialysis in such patients requires reduced heparinisation or regional heparinisation of the extra-corporeal dialysis circuit to reduce the risk of bleeding from the pericardium. Both asterixis and hiccoughing are signs of uraemic encephalopathy, which also indicates the need for dialysis but with less urgency than with pericarditis. Hyperkalaemia requires immediate treatment: if a patient is not anuric dialysis may not be required; insulin and dextrose infusion, calcium gluconate, correction of acidosis and salbutamol nebulisation remain the mainstay of immediate treatment of hyperkalaemia. Peripheral neuropathy may occur in chronic uraemia but is not a feature of acute renal failure unless caused by certain substances in overdose or exposure.

3.15   C: He takes atenolol for hypertension

Haemolytic disease of the newborn is the result of incompatibility of red cell antigens between mother and fetus; there is no association with uraemia occurring in later life. Drug history is an important part of the history in a patient with renal problems; in this scenario chronic analgesic usage and use of atenolol for hypertension are important factors. In addition to β-blockers, methylsergide (a constituent of migraine therapies) may cause retroperitoneal fibrosis, a cause of renal failure. Childhood haematuria may indicate a progressive glomerulonephritis or a familial renal disease such as Alport's syndrome. Chronic exposure to silica, in foundry workers, can lead to heavy metal-type interstitial nephritis or glomerulosclerosis.

3.16   E: The blood insulin level is disproportionately high for the blood glucose level

Of the given statements, only E is commonly seen. In chronic renal failure there is insulin resistance and so the insulin level is raised in proportion to the blood glucose level to maintain normoglycaemia. In childhood uraemia, acidosis is the most important contributor to growth retardation. Polyuria is common in moderate renal failure because of lack of urinary concentrating ability, partly due to relative insensitivity of the collecting ducts to ADH. Urinary calcium excretion is low in uraemia; hyperparathyroidism is common due primarily to deficient metabolism of vitamin D to its active form by the failing kidney. Control of hypertension stabilises GFR provided profound hypotension does not occur.

3.17   E: Retroperitoneal fibrosis by medial ureteric displacement on intravenous urograms

Renal obstruction is diagnosed by ultrasound; pressure studies may be required if the collecting system is dilated. Dehydration is itself a contraindication to performing intravenous urograms due to the increased risk of contrast nephropathy, particularly in diabetics, the elderly and arteriopaths; urograms will not aid diagnosis of dehydration. Coarse kidney scarring is caused by obstructive uropathy, papillary necrosis and renovascular disease in addition to reflux nephropathy. The diagnosis of retroperitoneal fibrosis is made by intravenous urograms; confirmation is made by biopsy of the peri-aortic mass seen on computed tomography (CT) or MRI. Associations with retroperitoneal fibrosis include drugs (β-blockers, methyldopa, bromocriptine and methylsergide) and carcinoid tumours. Large kidneys may indicate amyloidosis, diabetes or polycystic kidneys, so do not exclude parenchymal pathology.

3.18   E: The occurrence of renal vein thrombosis

Membranous glomerulonephritis accounts for 20–30% of adult nephrotic syndrome. It is associated with malignancy, autoimmune diseases and infections. On renal biopsy the common findings are thickened basement membrane with IgG and C3 subepithelial deposition. Between 5% and 10% of patients develop renal vein thrombosis and if albumin is persistently very low, anticoagulation is recommended. End-stage renal failure occurs in approximately one-third of patients but usually over a period of several years from diagnosis. Highly selective proteinuria is more likely in minimal-change glomerulonephritis which accounts for 75% of childhood nephrotic syndrome. If renal function deteriorates, treatment with cyclophosphamide and chlorambucil may be undertaken. IgM may be found in the mesangium in nephrotic syndrome as the mesangium acts as a 'scavenger' for filtered proteins but basement membrane deposition of IgM is not a characteristic feature of membranous glomerulonephritis.

3.19   A: Glomerular crescents may occur during episodes of macroscopic haematuria

In Europe, North America and Australia, IgA nephropathy is the most common form of glomerulonephritis. Only 15–20% of patients will eventually require dialysis. In common with all parenchymal renal disease, heavy proteinuria, eg more than 1g/day, implies a worse prognosis. Other poor prognostic factors include abnormal renal function at presentation and frequent episodes of macroscopic haematuria. Episodes of macroscopic haematuria often occur in conjunction with infection and are characterised histologically by glomerular crescents. Loin pain occurs at such times due to renal parenchymal swelling and not because of bleeding.

3.20   E: Renal amyloidosis

Any cause of nephrotic syndrome may be complicated by renal vein thrombosis, especially membranous glomerulonephritis. Causes of hyperviscosity, including severe dehydration and myeloma, may also be complicated by renal vein thrombosis. There are clotting derangements that occur in amyloidosis which predispose to renal vein thrombosis. Renal carcinoma may invade the renal veins which predisposes to thrombosis that may propagate into the inferior vena cava. Another risk factor for renal vein thrombosis is trauma to the vein, in particular cannulation.

3.21   B: Cystinosis

Noonan's syndrome is a hereditary form of hypertrophic cardiomyopathy; it is inherited in an autosomal dominant fashion and is not associated with any renal features. von Hippel–Lindau syndrome is also inherited in an autosomal dominant fashion and manifests as spinal and cerebellar haemangiomas, renal carcinomas and retinal angiomas. Childhood polycystic kidney disease has autosomal recessive inheritance; the gene is localised to chromosome 6 and end-stage renal failure develops early in childhood – prognosis is poor. Vesico-ureteric reflux has a familial predisposition and in some families is inherited as an autosomal dominant trait. Cystinosis is inherited in an autosomal recessive fashion; cardinal features are short stature, chronic renal failure, eye and cardiac disease; Fanconi's syndrome occurring with proximal renal tubular acidosis may be caused by cystinosis.

3.22   A: Age at presentation

Vesico-ureteric reflux often remains undiagnosed until presentation with chronic renal failure in adulthood. Evidence of urinary tract infection only occurs in approximately 40% of cases. Definitive investigation is a micturating cystourethrogram demonstrating reflux. Other useful investigations are intravenous urogram and radionuclide scanning; the kidneys are usually small and irregularly scarred. In some families there may be autosomal dominant inheritance of reflux disease. Once renal failure has occurred antireflux surgery is of limited benefit, except for symptomatic relief; antibiotics are indicated for urinary tract infections. ANCA antibodies are not associated with vesico-ureteric reflux. It is important to investigate whether ANCA antibodies are raised against myeloperoxidase or PR3, which are associated with renal disease, or are raised against other neutrophil antigens such as lactoferrin.

3.23   C: Normal chest X-ray

Constitutional symptoms such as fever and night sweats occur in less than 20% of patients with urinary tuberculosis (TB). Sterile pyuria and/or microscopic haematuria only occur in approximately 25% of cases. Tuberculous cystitis causes frequency, urgency and dysuria; occasionally, urge incontinence necessitates urinary diversion or a bladder augmentation operation. There are no radiological signs of pulmonary TB in approximately 60% of cases. Raised serum ACE levels are a non-specific finding more commonly associated with sarcoidosis but serum ACE is also raised in lymphoma, pulmonary TB, asbestosis and silicosis.

3.24   E: There is reduced ammonia formation despite a normal GFR

In distal renal tubular acidosis, the fundamental defect is a failure of hydrogen ion excretion into the urine. This means that there is reduced ammonia formation and, due to the lack of distal tubule hydrogen ion secretion, hypokalaemia occurs as potassium ions are secreted in exchange for sodium ions as sodium is reabsorbed. Nephrocalcinosis occurs in 70% of cases and while renal function is commonly preserved, renal tract calculi can lead to renal dysfunction. Most commonly, distal renal tubular acidosis is inherited in an autosomal dominant fashion. It is also associated with autoimmune disease (Sjögren's syndrome, chronic active hepatitis), drugs (lithium, amphotericin) and nephrocalcinosis due to other causes (hyperparathyroidism, medullary sponge kidney).

3.25   D: Omeprazole

Of these drugs, omeprazole is the safest to use in renal failure as its clearance is not affected by decreasing renal function. However, in patients who have received a renal transplant and are taking ciclosporin care is needed as omeprazole often leads to an increase in ciclosporin levels. Oxytetracycline exacerbates uraemia by increasing urea generation; all tetracyclines except doxycycline have this effect. Mesalazine can provoke interstitial nephritis through its sulphonamide component. Both ibuprofen and lisinopril may compromise renal perfusion in circumstances of volume depletion such as hypotension due to cardiac failure or in elderly patients with an intercurrent illness. ACE inhibitors and angiotensin-II receptor antagonists must be used with caution in uraemia; they do have an antiproteinuria effect which may slow the decline in renal function in addition to their hypotensive effect.

3.26   E: It is often associated with eosinophilia

Cholesterol emboli to the kidneys usually arise from an atheromatous aorta, and may be triggered by instrumentation (eg arteriography). They are found at autopsy in 17% of patients over 60 years of age, although they may be subclinical. The crystals usually lodge in arteries of diameter 150–300 mm, so complete renal infarction resulting in loin pain and haematuria is rare. There is typically evidence of microinfarcts elsewhere on the lower extremities, such as livedo reticularis and gangrenous toes. Leucocytosis, eosinophilia and reduced C3 are typical but not invariable findings.

3.27   B: Pulsed methylprednisolone may be used in treatment

Hepatitis C causes an immune complex-mediated membranoproliferative glomerulonephritis. The immunoglobulins are not cold agglutinins (antibodies causing agglutination of erythrocytes in the cold peripheries of the body), but cryoglobulins (types II and III mixed). Cryoglobulins are immunoglobulins that reversibly precipitate in the cold. One-third of patients exhibit spontaneous renal remission. Interferon-α is used in treatment; pulsed methylprednisolone and plasma exchange are also of value.

3.28   E: Mesangial widening, basement membrane thickening and capillary obliteration

Hyaline thrombi are found in monoclonal immunoglobulin deposition diseases, SLE and thrombotic microangiopathies. The typical changes of membranous glomerulonephritis include capillary thickening, and spike- and-chain appearance of the basement membrane. Mesangial hypercellularity is seen in the proliferative glomerulopathies: post-streptococcal, mesangiocapillary, IgA/Henoch–Schönheim purpura, SLE, vasculitides, endocarditis. Green birefringence on staining with Congo red is a feature of amyloidosis.

3.29   E: Normal parathyroid hormone levels

The 1,25-dihydroxycholecalciferol is low or normal, not (as would be expected for the degree of hypophosphataemia) elevated. There is renal phosphate wasting, but glycosuria and aminoaciduria are absent. The condition is X-linked but females may be affected by lyonisation.

3.30 B: Gastric ulceration is partly attributable to increased rate of *H. pylori* carriage

Cardiovascular death is the most important cause of death following transplantation. The risk of malignancy is much increased after transplantation; in rarer tumours the risk may be increased by a factor of 1000.

Another predisposing risk factor for gastric ulceration is prednisolone therapy.

With regard to infective complications, reverse barrier nursing is now considered unnecessary. A CMV-negative recipient should not receive a kidney from a CMV-positive donor, due to the risk of overwhelming infection (70–80% infection rate; 2% mortality in patients with disseminated disease). However, a CMV-positive recipient could receive a CMV-negative kidney. *Pneumocystis* infection typically occurs at 2–4 months.

3.31 C: Fluid intake should be 2–3 litres per day

Patients with severe renal impairment usually require fluid restriction in order to avoid peripheral oedema, pulmonary oedema and hypertension. However, in moderate renal impairment, it is usually important to drink 2–3 litres per day, in order to excrete the obligatory osmolar load (there is impairment of urinary concentration). There is evidence that moderate protein restriction may help slow progression of chronic renal failure, but severe protein restriction is likely to result in malnutrition and is mainly used to attenuate the symptoms of uraemia in patients unsuitable for dialysis. Patients with chronic renal failure are at increased risk of vascular disease; cholesterol intake needs to be controlled carefully. Patients on a phosphate-restriction diet need to limit their intake of dairy products.

3.32 A: Haemodialysis following death cap mushroom ingestion does not affect mortality despite good toxin removal

Peritoneal dialysis is less effective than haemodialysis at toxin removal, and is only indicated where haemodialysis is technically impossible. Highly protein-bound toxins such as the tricyclics are not well removed by haemodialysis. Indications for haemodialysis in salicylate poisoning include coma, convulsions and acute renal failure. Use of bicarbonate buffer is mandatory, as acetate will exacerbate the metabolic acidosis. Death cap mushroom toxicity is not amenable to haemodialysis due to rapid and irreversible end-organ damage.

3.33   C: HIV-associated nephropathy typically presents with nephrotic-range proteinuria

Renal involvement is rare (3% of autopsies of AIDS patients). The typical histological feature of HIV-associated nephropathy is focal or global capillary collapse. It may respond to zidovudine. The natural history is rapid progression to end-stage renal failure. Other features of HIV infection include hyponatraemia, hyperkalaemia and hypocalcaemia.

3.34   D: Penicillamine

Penicillamine works by converting cystine to cysteine-penicillamine, which is 50 times more soluble, hence reducing crystallisation. It should be used in conjunction with a high fluid intake. Alkalisation of the urine is theoretically beneficial, but does not appear to be clinically useful. Cysteamine may be used in the treatment of cystinosis.

3.35   C: Ibuprofen

Thiazides reduce urinary calcium excretion and may be useful in management of idiopathic hypercalciuria.

Corticosteroids are used in the treatment of sarcoidosis, which is associated with calculi formation.

Cholestyramine reduces urinary oxalate excretion in the case of enteric hyperoxaluria.

Pyridoxine may be useful in reducing urinary oxalate excretion in idiopathic hyperoxaluria.

3.36   E: Dipstick urinalysis and microscopy

The patient has rhabdomyolysis following the muscle damage caused by his prolonged convulsion. The low calcium, and markedly elevated potassium, creatinine and phosphate are highly suggestive of this diagnosis. Dipstick urinalysis will test positive for blood (due to the myoglobinuria), but urine microscopy will not demonstrate haematuria. Renal biopsy would confirm the diagnosis more definitively.

3.37   B: Anti-glomerular basement membrane disease

The other causes of reduced CH50 in glomerulonephritis are shunt nephritis, type I mesangiocapillary glomerulonephritis, and infective endocarditis.

3.38   A: Adenoma sebaceum in a patient with microscopic haematuria

Accelerated or malignant hypertension, indicated fundoscopically by grade 3 or 4 changes, may be an aetiological factor in renal failure, but hypertension is of course also an important consequence of renal failure. Adenoma sebaceum (facial angiofibromas) is a typical finding in tuberose sclerosis, a condition characterised by bilateral renal angiomyolipomas and cysts. Deep vein thrombosis is a complication of the nephrotic syndrome. Cushing's syndrome is not typically associated with any renal disease.

Up to 90% of patients with partial lipodystrophy develop progressive glomerulonephritis, most usually mesangiocapillary glomerulonephritis type II. A serum creatinine of 150 µmol/l with normal urinary sediment is an unlikely presentation of this condition.

3.39   A: Infection two weeks ago with an α-haemolytic streptococcus

Post-streptococcal glomerulonephritis is associated with group A β-haemolytic streptococcus. The condition typically occurs 10 to 14 days after upper respiratory tract infection, or three weeks after a skin infection. It typically affects children aged three to eight years, boys more than girls. A quarter of patients have normal renal function at presentation and 10% have no elevation of ASOT. The proteinuria is typically less than 2 g in 24 hours.

3.40   A: Eclampsia can occur without previous hypertension

Korotkoff phase V may not occur in pregnancy, so it is important to use phase IV. Blood pressure falls in the first trimester, reaches a nadir in the mid-trimester, and by term is comparable to non-pregnant blood pressure. This physiological fall is due to reduced vascular resistance, both by vasodilatation, and later due to the uteroplacental circulation. Cardiac output increases by about 40%. The accepted threshold for physiological proteinuria is 0.3 g/24 hour. The risk of pre-eclampsia is 15 times greater for the first pregnancy than the second. Eclampsia occurs without any recognised pre-eclampsia in around 20% of cases.

3.41   C: Severe hyperphosphataemia is a contraindication to the administration of 1,25-hydroxy-vitamin D

The desferrioxamine stimulation test is used to diagnose aluminium overload, which may occur in haemodialysis patients, and is an important cause of renal bone disease.

Cheese is high in phosphate, which should be restricted in renal bone disease. (It is also high in fat, and a major cause of mortality in renal patients is vascular disease.) Phosphate binders must be taken with food, as they bind dietary phosphate. It is important that the phosphate is well controlled before calcitriol is prescribed, otherwise there is the risk of extra-skeletal calcification due to an elevated calcium-phosphate product.

Parathyroidectomy may be necessary in cases of severe tertiary hyper-parathyroidism.

3.42 A: Urinary protein excretion of 3 g/l, in conjunction with microscopic haematuria, may be attributable to strenuous exercise

Pathological levels of proteinuria are a reflection of (a) glomerular pathology, (b) elevated plasma protein levels (overflow proteinuria), or (c) tubular damage (eg Fanconi's syndrome). Orthostatic proteinuria disappears during recumbency.

Microalbuminuria is defined as proteinuria greater than the upper limit of normal (150 mg/24 h) but less than 100 mg/l (threshold for dipstick positivity).

In young adults, the main causes of nephrosis are minimal-change disease, focal segmental glomerulosclerosis, proliferative glomerulonephritides, and Henoch–Schönlein disease. Membranous glomerulonephritis is more commonly seen in older patients, due to its association with malignancy.

3.43 C: A 60-year-old man who developed type 1 DM 43 years ago

Type 1 DM

After development of diabetes, there is a lag period of about five years when development of nephropathy is rare. Thereafter, the annual incidence of the complication increases to a peak of 3% per year 15–17 years after development of diabetes. Patients who have had the disease for more than 35 years have a low risk of developing nephropathy.

Type 2 DM

Unlike type 1, the incidence of nephropathy rises steadily with time. The patient described in D is likely to have had undetected diabetes for some time: such patients may present with, or rapidly develop, retinopathy and nephropathy. There is considerable racial heterogeneity with regard to incidence of nephropathy. Japanese and Pima Indians have a cumulative incidence of 50% after 20 years of diabetes, compared with 25% for Caucasians.

3.44 A: Hypercalcaemia

The central feature of haemolytic uraemic syndrome is endothelial injury with platelet adhesion. There is an intravascular haemolytic anaemia, with a fall in haptoglobin, elevated reticulocyte count, thrombocytopenia and neutrophilia. There is usually hyponatraemia.

3.45   A: Acute renal failure in childhood

Peritoneal dialysis is often the modality of choice in childhood. It presents fewer technical difficulties than haemodialysis and the peritoneal membrane is functionally more efficient than in adults. Peritoneal dialysis has a very limited role in removal of poisons.

Relative contraindications to peritoneal dialysis include :

*   any previous condition or procedure likely to have caused significant peritoneal scarring

*   any condition where the splinting of the diaphragm by the dialysate is likely to be deleterious

*   factors making the patient unable to perform the exchanges safely (only relevant for chronic dialysis ie CAPD), such as dementia, poor hygiene, severe arthritis

*   pre-existing malnutrition, as peritoneal dialysis causes continuous protein loss.

3.46   B: The net insensible water loss is approximately 0.2 l/day

A clinically relevant question! It is important to be able to estimate the insensible losses of a patient accurately. In a normothermic patient, they will be approximately 0.5 l/day. However, this will rise significantly if the patient is pyrexial. Massive fluid volumes can be tolerated acutely in the normal patient. The hyponatraemia seen in psychogenic polydipsia is probably related to impairment of free water excretion.

3.47   A: Cardiac/vascular

Anyone who answered B or E must have little faith in the nephrological service in this country! Malignancy is an important complication of transplantation. Infection is the second greatest cause of death, reflecting both the increased susceptibility of these patients to infection, and the instrumentation they require. However, vascular (including cardiac) causes of death account for 40–50% of all deaths in patients on dialysis. This is partly due to some of the conditions which result in ESRF (diabetes, renal artery disease) and to the increased number of elderly patients now receiving dialysis. However, renal failure itself increases the incidence of atherosclerotic disease, due to hypertension, lipid abnormalities, anaemia, and altered vessel wall characteristics.

3.48   E: 1 g/day of proteinuria would be expected with haematuria due to a bladder malignancy

A family history of microscopic haematuria may provide a clue to Alport's syndrome or benign familial haematuria. Only major haematuria (> 50 ml/24 h) allows enough protein loss into the urine to give a positive result on dipstick testing. Presence of significant proteinuria should point the clinician firmly towards a renal origin.

3.49   C: Continuous veno-venous haemofiltration

In order to confirm a diagnosis of hepatorenal syndrome over pre-renal azotaemia, it is often necessary to ensure that there is no reversibility in response to a fluid challenge, and/or to measure the central venous pressure as an estimate of vascular filling. However, once the diagnosis has been made, fluid and sodium restriction are crucial. Whereas orthotopic liver transplantation may be life-saving, the kidneys are normal, and do not require transplantation.

Although the renin-angiotensin system is implicated in the pathogenesis of hepatorenal syndrome, trials of the use of ACE inhibitors have resulted in severe hypotension.

Some form of dialysis is often necessary to prevent life-threatening fluid overload, and to permit fluid administration of bicarbonate or hyperalimentation regimes. However, patients often exhibit too much cardiovascular instability to tolerate haemodialysis, and continuous veno-venous haemofiltration may be used instead.

3.50   B: Liver ultrasonography of patient

Neonatally, the two conditions are clinically indistinguishable. They are also indistinguishable on renal ultrasonography. Renal ultrasound on the parents will only be conclusive, in the case of a negative examination, if the parents are over the age of 30. There is no indication for IVP or renal biopsy. However, hepatic ultrasound should demonstrate biliary dysgenesis in the case of the recessive condition. Ultimately, genetic studies are most likely to be definitive.

REVISION CHECKLISTS

ENDOCRINOLOGY: REVISION CHECKLIST

Diabetes and glycaemic control

- [ ] Diabetes
- [ ] Hypoglycaemia
- [ ] Glycosylated haemoglobin
- [ ] Hepatic gluconeogenesis
- [ ] Insulinoma

Adrenal disease

- [ ] Cushing's syndrome
- [ ] Addison's disease
- [ ] Congenital adrenal hyperplasia
- [ ] ACTH action
- [ ] Conn's disease

Thyroid disease

- [ ] Thyroxine action/metabolism TFTs
- [ ] Thyroid cancer/nodule
- [ ] Graves' disease/exophthalmos
- [ ] Hypothyroidism

Parathyroid disease/Calcium

- [ ] PTH/hyperparathyroidism
- [ ] Calcitonin

Pituitary disease

- [ ] Acromegaly
- [ ] Chromophobe adenoma
- [ ] Hyperprolactinaemia
- [ ] Hypopituitarism
- [ ] Pituitary hormones

Miscellaneous

☐ Polycystic ovarian syndrome/infertility

☐ SIADH

☐ Short stature

☐ Weight gain/Prader–Willi syndrome

☐ Endocrine changes in anorexia

☐ Hirsutism

☐ Hormone physiology (including pregnancy)

☐ Sweating

GASTROENTEROLOGY: REVISION CHECKLIST

Liver disease

☐ Chronic liver disease
☐ Jaundice
☐ Primary biliary cirrhosis
☐ Gilbert's syndrome
☐ Hepatic mass/subphrenic abscess
☐ Alcohol and the liver
☐ Portal vein thrombosis

Small bowel disease/malabsorption

☐ Coeliac disease
☐ Malabsorption/protein-losing enteropathy
☐ Cholera toxin/gastroenteritis
☐ Carcinoid syndrome
☐ Whipple's disease
    (see also 'Crohn's disease' below)

Large bowel disorders

☐ Crohn's disease
☐ Ulcerative colitis/colonic carcinoma
☐ Irritable bowel syndrome
☐ Diarrhoea
☐ Inflammatory bowel disease – general
☐ Pseudomembranous colitis

Oesophageal disease

☐ Gastro-oesophageal reflux/tests
☐ Achalasia
☐ Dysphagia/oesophageal tumour
☐ Oesophageal chest pain

Stomach and pancreas

- ☐ Acute pancreatitis
- ☐ Gastric acid secretion
- ☐ Persistent vomiting
- ☐ Stomach cancer

Miscellaneous

- ☐ GI tract bleeding
- ☐ Abdominal X-ray
- ☐ GI hormones
- ☐ Physiology of absorption
- ☐ Recurrent abdominal pain
- ☐ Gall bladder disease

NEPHROLOGY: REVISION CHECKLIST

Nephrotic syndrome/related glomerulonephritis

- [ ] Nephrotic syndrome
- [ ] Membranous glomerulonephritis
- [ ] Minimal-change disease
- [ ] Hypocomplementaemia and glomerulonephritis
- [ ] Renal vein thrombosis
- [ ] Acute glomerulonephritis
- [ ] SLE nephritis

Renal failure

- [ ] Acute renal failure
- [ ] Acute versus chronic
- [ ] Chronic renal failure
- [ ] Haemolytic-uraemic syndrome
- [ ] Rhabdomyolysis
- [ ] Anaemia in renal failure
- [ ] Contrast nephropathy

Urinary abnormalities

- [ ] Macroscopic haematuria
- [ ] Discoloration of the urine
- [ ] Nocturia
- [ ] Polyuria

Basic renal physiology

- [ ] Normal renal physiology/function
- [ ] Water excretion/urinary concentration
- [ ] Serum creatinine

Miscellaneous

- ☐ Distal renal tubular acidosis
- ☐ Renal papillary necrosis
- ☐ Diabetic nephropathy
- ☐ Analgesic nephropathy
- ☐ Polycystic kidney disease
- ☐ Renal calculi
- ☐ Renal osteodystrophy
- ☐ Retroperitoneal fibrosis
- ☐ Steroid therapy in renal disease

INDEX

Locators refer to question number.

Nephrology

PASTEST BOOKS FOR MRCP PART 1

MRCP 1 Pocket Book Series
Further titles in this range:

Book 1:	Cardiology, Haematology, Respiratory	1 901198 75 8
Book 2:	Basic Sciences, Neurology, Psychiatry	1 901198 80 4
Book 4:	Clinical Pharmacology, Infectious Diseases,	
	Immunology, Rheumatology	1 901198 90 1

Essential Revision Notes for MRCP: Revised Edition
Philip Kalra   1 901198 59 6
A definitive guide to revision for the MRCP examination that offers 19 chapters of informative material necessary to gain a successful exam result.

MRCP 1: Best of Five Practice Papers
Khalid Binymin   1 901198 88 X
Four practice papers with 100 questions in each. Excellent up-to-date clinical scenarios.

MRCP 1 'Best of Five' Multiple Choice Revision Book
Khalid Binymin   1 901198 57 X
This book features subject-based chapters ensuring all topics are fully covered.

MRCP 1 300 Best of Five
Geraint Rees   1 901198 97 9
300 brand new 'Best of Five' questions with excellent clinical scenarios encountered in everyday hospital practice.

MRCP 1: Best of Five Key Topic Summaries: Third Edition
Stephen Waring & Paul O'Neill   1 904627 05 6
Subject-based chapters in 'Best of Five' format with excellent clinical scenarios.

Essential Lists for MRCP
Stuart McPherson   1 901198 58 8
The lists contained in this book offer a compilation of clinical, diagnostic, investigative and prognostic features of the symptoms and diseases that cover the whole spectrum of general medicine. It is invaluable for MRCP Part 1 AND Part 2.

MRCP 1 Multiple True/False Revision Book
Philip Kalra   1 901198 95 2
600 multiple true/false questions in subject-based chapters and three 'test yourself' practice exams to give experience of exam fomat.

MCQs in Basic Medical Sciences for MRCP Part 1
Philippa Easterbrook   1 906896 34 7
300 exam-based MCQs focusing on basic sciences with expanded teaching notes.

PASTEST – DEDICATED TO YOUR SUCCESS

PasTest has been publishing books for doctors for over 30 years. Our extensive experience means that we are always one step ahead when it comes to knowledge of current trends and content of the Royal College exams.

We use only the best authors and lecturers, many of whom are Consultants and Royal College Examiners, which enables us to tailor our books and courses to meet your revision needs. We incorporate feedback from candidates to ensure that our books are continually improved.

This commitment to quality ensures that students who buy a PasTest book or attend a PasTest course achieve successful exam results.

Delivery to your Door

With a busy lifestyle, nobody enjoys walking to the shops for something that may or may not be in stock. Let us take away the hassle and deliver direct to your door. We will despatch your book within 24 hours of receiving your order. We also offer free delivery on books for medical students to UK addresses.

How to Order:

💻 **www.pastest.co.uk**

   To order books safely and securely online, shop at our website.

☎ **Telephone: +44 (0)1565 752000**

📠 **Fax: +44 (0)1565 650264**

✉ **PasTest Ltd, FREEPOST, Knutsford, WA16 7BR.**